S0-BDL-119

DISCARD

# IN VIVO

*The Cultural Mediations of Biomedical Science*

PHILLIP THURTLE and ROBERT MITCHELL, Series Editors

IN VIVO: THE CULTURAL MEDIATIONS OF BIOMEDICAL SCIENCE is dedicated to the interdisciplinary study of the medical and life sciences, with a focus on the scientific and cultural practices used to process data, model knowledge, and communicate about biomedical science. Through historical, artistic, media, social, and literary analysis, books in the series seek to understand and explain the key conceptual issues that animate and inform biomedical developments.

*The Transparent Body: A Cultural Analysis of Medical Imaging*
by José Van Dijck

*Generating Bodies and Gendered Selves: The Rhetoric of Reproduction in Early Modern England*
by Eve Keller

*The Emergence of Genetic Rationality: Space, Time, and Information in American Biological Science, 1870–1920*
by Phillip Thurtle

*Bits of Life: Feminist Studies of Media, Biocultures, and Technoscience*
edited by Anneke Smelik and Nina Lykke

*HIV Interventions: Biomedicine and the Traffic between Information and Flesh*
by Marsha Rosengarten

# HIV Interventions

*Biomedicine and the Traffic between Information and Flesh*

MARSHA ROSENGARTEN

UNIVERSITY OF WASHINGTON PRESS

*Seattle and London*

Copyright © 2009 by the University of Washington Press
Designed by Thomas Eykemans
Printed in the United States of America
15 14 13 12 11 10 09    5 4 3 2 1

UNIVERSITY OF WASHINGTON PRESS
PO Box 50096
Seattle, WA 98145–5096, USA
*www.washington.edu/uwpress*

All rights reserved. No part of this publication may be reproduced or transmitted in any form or by any means, electronic or mechanical, including photocopy, recording, or any information storage or retrieval system, without permission in writing from the publisher.

LIBRARY OF CONGRESS CATALOGING-IN-PUBLICATION DATA
Rosengarten, Marsha.
HIV interventions : biomedicine and the traffic between information and flesh / Marsha Rosengarten.
    p. ; cm. — (In vivo)
"A Samuel and Althea Stroum book."
Includes bibliographical references and index.
ISBN 978-0-295-98959-4 (hbk. : alk. paper)
ISBN 978-0-295-98942-6 (pbk. : alk. paper)
1. AIDS (Disease)—Social aspects. I. Title. II. Series: In vivo (Seattle, Wash.)
[DNLM: 1. HIV Infections—prevention & control. 2. HIV Infections—psychology. 3. Health Knowledge, Attitudes, Practice. 4. Health Promotion. 5. Information Theory. WC 503.6 R812h 2009]
RA643.8.R67 2009
362.196'9792—dc22                                          2009013453

The paper used in this publication is acid-free and 90 percent recycled from at least 50 percent post-consumer waste. It meets the minimum requirements of American National Standard for Information Sciences—Permanence of Paper for Printed Library Materials, ANSI z39.48-1984.

*for those who live with the epidemic*

# Contents

# Acknowledgments

T HIS BOOK BEGAN SOMETIME AGO WITHOUT MY REALIZING IT, WHILE I
was working at the National Centre in HIV Social Research, University
of New South Wales, with an energetic team of committed staff led by Susan
Kippax, who remains an inspiration to me in many ways. Kane Race was
one of the first people I met there and I am deeply indebted to him as a col-
league and a friend. I thank him most especially for the erudite feedback he
provided on earlier drafts. Many evenings were spent with Dean Murphy
as we shared a flat and together tried to decipher the uncanny way HIV
prevention and treatment can undermine each other. I am very grateful to
him for pointing me to material that invariably proved relevant in subtle
and important ways. My research in the UK draws significantly from my
experience of working with John Imrie at Mortimer Market Clinic and for
this I also thank Ian Weller, the staff, and patients. The content reflects the
dual perspective on the epidemic I have gained by my move from Australia
to the United Kingdom.

Throughout I have been immensely lucky to have the friendship of a
number of very smart and generous thinkers. I value very much the intense
and stimulating discussions I have had with Ros Diprose and with Susie
MacLean and the support and encouragement I have received from Jane
Becker, Carla Drago, Harriet Grahame, Diane Hamer, Caroline Lawrance,
Niamh Stephenson, Nicole Vitellone, Catherine Waldby, and Elizabeth Wilson. At Goldsmiths, I especially want to thank Lisa Adkins, Vikki Bell, Mariam Fraser, Celia Lury, Mike Michael, and Nirmal Puwar. I want to add that
I feel very fortunate to be part of a department that has taken such a leading
role in the theoretical work that I have found so valuable.

There are many others in the HIV field, plus, most important, those I
have interviewed over the years—without whom this book could not have
developed. In particular I want to thank Jamie Dunbar and Mark Chester

for entrusting me to reproduce their work in the context of my own account of the epidemic and to the AIDS Council of New South Wales (ACON) for allowing me to reproduce David McDiarmid's poster, which hangs above my desk and is a constant reminder that "in your face" innovation can be an effective intervention.

The editorial advice provided by my editors Jacqueline Ettinger, Robert Mitchell, and Phillip Thurtle has been immensely important throughout, as has the very valuable feedback of two reviewers in the last stages.

Finally I want to thank Cath Le Couteur for the many things she has brought to this book. Most remarkable for me has been her astonishing ability to discern what matters in the minefield of biomedical innovation and her own personal generosity in enabling some of the wanted benefits that can follow.

# HIV Interventions

*Biomedicine and the Traffic between Information and Flesh*

# 1

# INTRODUCTION:
# HIV, INFORMATION, AND FLESH

> Information, so the story goes, exists between elements, whereas bodies are
> the elements themselves. Information underwrites signs and syntax, whereas
> the flesh is the medium of cells and organs. Information, in short, operates
> through the metaphysics of absence, whereas bodies depend on the meta-
> physics of presence.
>
> —Robert Mitchell and Phillip Thurtle, *Data Made Flesh*

SINCE THE LATE 1990S, IT HAS BEEN APPARENT THAT A COCKTAIL OF antiretroviral drugs (ARVs), designed to intercept the replication of the human immunodeficiency virus (HIV) in vivo, can significantly halt or, at least, forestall the otherwise almost inevitable progression to Acquired Immunodeficiency Syndrome (AIDS).[1] In epidemiological terms, the most outstanding change since the early years of the AIDS epidemic has been the statistical decline in the number of people with HIV who go on to develop AIDS.[2] This advance has been so significant that AIDS is no longer the consequence of HIV that it once was. Indeed, it is possible to claim that as a result of ARVs, HIV and AIDS have become "decoupled," so to speak, at least at the present time.[3] However, this decoupling needs to be viewed as part of a dynamic process whereby both the nature of HIV *and* its treatment and prevention are altered through what we might view as a mutually affective process.

There can be no doubt that—for those with full access to ARVs—living with HIV in the post-ARV period is preferable to living with HIV in the pre-ARV period, though it is worth remembering that, in our global context, more than 70 percent of people infected with HIV are without full access to

ARVs.[4] Yet even for HIV-positive individuals with access to ARVs, life with HIV has not necessarily become easier, and the terrain of treating and living with HIV remains, for many, immensely complicated and distressing. While the increasing array of specialist drugs and diagnostics to deal with HIV has brought new knowledge of the virus and the means for reducing its chances of replicating, the drugs and diagnostics are also "productive" in the sense that they generate new medical and prevention concerns. Thus, more than twelve years after the announcement that a combination of antiretrovirals can significantly delay AIDS, mounting data suggests that there are now a host of unwanted drug side effects and these extend across the disciplinary biological/flesh and social/information split.[5] Although it is likely that the well-documented unwanted effects identified under the heading of "biological" will be reduced with new drug formulations, I have elected to use these unwanted effects and those of a said "social" nature to highlight the generative work of intervention. I suggest that if we are to understand the challenge of HIV, we must understand our field of inquiry—here identified as efforts to deal with HIV from a scientific paradigm—as consisting not simply of the virus but of the virus already entangled in attempts to know and intervene in its destructive course.

## INFORMATION AS FLESH

To understand what emerges in association with a virus conceptualized through the highly sophisticated technologies of immunology, virology, and epidemiology and targeted by ARVs, I contend that we must be willing to collapse the apparent distinction between "information" and "flesh" that implicitly guides many scientific and policy approaches to biotechnologies in general, and HIV and AIDS in particular. As one brief illustration of how the distinction may function as an obstruction to more effective intervention, it is worth considering current debate about whether widespread publicity of an HIV prophylaxis to prevent the onset of HIV infection after possible exposure—"post-exposure prophylaxis" or PEP—will undermine a culture of safe-sex practices and, paradoxically, increase infection.[6] Underpinning this framing of PEP is, on the one hand, a human subject conceived as a source and enactment of "information" or sign with the capacity to act and, on the other "flesh" hand, a biotechnology (PEP) and human body within which PEP may or may not prevent infection. On the basis of the distinction, attention focuses on the human subject and the question that arises is whether "he" can be trusted to sustain a practice of safe sex with knowledge of the technology or, alternately, whether the technology should be withheld.[7] Besides the normative dimensions of this summation whereby the subject is already presumed to possess the potential to go awry, the evaluation is of concern because it means a far more pressing question of how to advance prevention slips from view.[8] By assuming a hard and fast distinction between information and flesh, biotechnologies remain as no more than "tools" that can give rise to "good" or "bad" effects and the assemblage in which they have an agentive role passes without interrogation.

In contrast, and as my title already suggests, I propose we consider biotechnologies as active in the materialization of the object that they are more conventionally understood to identify and/or intervene in. Rather than making a hard and fast distinction between "information" and "flesh," I suggest we instead seek to illuminate those dynamic processes that involve a coextensive relation between information and flesh: that is, processes through which what initially seems to be "information" turns out to transform that which we know as "flesh" or, conversely, flesh turns out to have informational effects.[9] This by no means involves denying the realness of HIV or the welcome changes that can be attributed to scientific intervention for those living with HIV. Rather, it is to recognize a more extensive, relational, and generative process than is apparent in conventional thinking about intervention.[10]

The peculiar nature of the virus that is at the center of the field of HIV research and intervention already highlights the need for such a collapse between concepts of information and flesh. Characterized as a retrovirus, HIV is simultaneously information, material, and materialized in its expression:

> Retroviruses were so named because they reverse what seemed to be the normal flow of genetic information. In cells the genetic material is DNA; when genes are expressed, the DNA is first transcribed into messenger RNA, which then serves as the template for the production of proteins. The genes of a retrovirus are encoded in RNA; before they can be expressed the RNA must be converted into DNA. Only then are the viral genes transcribed and translated into proteins in the usual sequence.[11]

According to scientific description, HIV is a movement in information as flesh. The collapse of the presumed distinction between information and flesh, as the science of HIV suggests, wreaks immense destruction as code alters code—yet this is code that remains, at the same time, flesh.[12] The process or traffic of genetic transcription, known as HIV, is one of debilitation as well as replication through transfer. In a simplified immunological account, this rewriting leads to more and more viral RNA becoming inscribed into the DNA of more and more cells.[13] The effect is that necessary cells are gradually killed off by the rewriting of their working codes.

As I explore in this book, this confusion of information and flesh also occurs, albeit in a different way, in the interventions—including ARVs—to prevent AIDS within an individual body or to limit the transmission of HIV across bodies. That is to say, the devising and implementing of diagnostic tests and pharmaceutical drugs to arrest the virus can be viewed as a dynamic process that cannot be held to a distinction between information and flesh.[14] For those working in the prevention field, the "traffic" in information as flesh may be recognizable in alterations to risk understandings and practices, which have taken place with antiretroviral drug suppression of viral replication. For those in the medical field, the traffic may be further recognizable in the appearance of new infections bearing the effects of drug-insensitive virus, that is, drug-resistant virus.[15] The central aim of this book is therefore to review the work of HIV biomedical interventions to show the part they play and the ways in which they are altered yet, also, ethically implicated in the manifest challenges of the HIV/AIDS epidemic, nearly thirty years since the virus was first identified.

## INFORMATION AS FLESH IN THE HISTORY OF HIV/AIDS ACTIVISM

While framing questions of HIV intervention in terms of "information as flesh" is perhaps unusual in recent analyses of the work of ARVs, this framing nevertheless has antecedents in critiques of science that commenced around the time of the original identification of HIV/AIDS. Even prior to the identification of HIV/AIDS, there was within the social sciences and some strands of philosophy a longstanding debate about the privileged status and work of the natural sciences.[16] However, the way in which HIV/AIDS emerged as an epidemic of death, fueled by a thinly veiled abhorrence of those already marked as different, mobilized cultural theorists and spurred communities into action against not just the "God's eye" stance of science but also the fallacies that are bound up with this stance.[17] As Cindy Patton noted early in the epidemic, one of the consequences of hegemonic science as an arbiter of true or correct knowledge is the foreclosure on "the exchange of crucial forms of information about transmission interruption both within and between communities."[18] Her work from a pre-ARVs period continues to resonate owing to its many insights into the workings of science. In 1990 she pointed to the political effects of a logic that reduces complex life phenomena to behaviors to be judged and regulated and, in doing so, exposed how such a logic contradicts the objective manner that it presupposes:

> In AIDS medical science, the body becomes a screen or agar plate on which disease is in play. . . . Diagnostic medicine abstracts the symptoms from the body to produce a totalizing explanation with a single or primary cause, a pathology. Because the immune system, understood metaphorically, transcends the place of the body, the abstraction "AIDS" folds back to correspond exactly to the space of the body. The virus is lost and, metaphorically speaking, the homosexual/prostitute/African/injecting-drug-user/hemophiliac body becomes AIDS.[19]

With hindsight it is not difficult to see that, pre-ARVs, HIV science was held back by cultural assumptions about who was infected by HIV and how they became infected. This is most explicit in the initial naming of HIV/AIDS as Gay Related Immune Deficiency or GRID. Although the term never became official, its proposal in the early 1980s exemplifies the way in which science is always entangled with what is seen as its other, that is, culture.[20] GRID was materialized through a mix of phenomena, including laboratory-based science, clinical observation, and the exercise of an epidemiological gaze, which sought to explain the presence of anomalous infections in a cultural category of young, otherwise healthy males who had had anal intercourse with other men. This category of persons was soon noted to share what, mistakenly, seemed to those in the observing medical and epidemiological professions an important characteristic in itself: same-sex desire.[21] By connecting a tragic terminal disease to non-heteronormative sexual desire, the significance of practices rather than desire as the means of transmission was lost and the myth of objective observation reigned. While scientists, epidemiologists, and clinicians worked hard to provide what they believed was a purely scientific explanation for a terminal infection, they provided the ground for a moral panic that reflected and aided stigma, discrimination, and exclusion. Most explicitly, HIV—whether termed GRID or HIV—bore a prior investment in an already pathologized gay sexuality, an investment in a thinly guised moral claim of gay sexuality as not "right" and made this the explanation for illness. Consistent with Patton's observation, cited above, yet more drawn to what was characterized at the time as homophobia, Paula Treichler observed that:

> Whatever else it may be, AIDS is a story, or multiple stories, read to a surprising extent from a text that does not exist: the body of the male homosexual. It is a text people so want—need—to read that they have gone so far as to write it themselves. AIDS is a nexus where multiple meanings, stories, and discourses intersect and overlap, reinforce, and subvert one another. Yet clearly this mysterious male homosexual text has figured centrally in generating what I call here an epidemic of signification.[22]

Although science had found that transmission was caused by the exchange of bodily fluids and this meant that sexual, ethnic, or racial identity categories were not the basis for risk, this important distinction was effectively sidelined. Contributing to critical scholarly work on the social construction of HIV/AIDS and especially in the United States, Julia Epstein noted that "[u]nless you can prove that you are an 'innocent victim,' something must have been wrong with you from the start for you to have contracted this disease."[23] The implication of choice as a factor in how a person acquired the virus was immensely significant. For it implied that those who have HIV—as a result of activities not related to medical culpability such as a contaminated blood transfusion—were guilty and therefore responsible because they "knowingly" engaged in wrongful behavior.[24] In the context informing Epstein's writing, the explanatory narratives she identifies—sexual volition, pleasure, and substance use—functioned to reassure an invented "general population" that they were safe. At the same time, by appropriating the pathologizing of same sex desire and conflating this with HIV infection, the rhetoric functioned to construct a "general population" from whom the vast majority of people with HIV were excluded.[25] This practice was especially rife in the United States in the absence of government challenge. Indeed, it can be argued that the conflation of disease and identity, with its particular exclusionary construction of risk, was directly responsible for the growth of the epidemic and its extension into different sexual communities in the United States, compared to countries such as Australia, the United Kingdom, and Canada, where the governments did intervene.[26] As this account of the early history of the HIV/AIDS epidemic suggests, the "informational" and "fleshy" aspects of this epidemic bled into one another, as "information" on HIV/AIDS constructed, pathologized, and, in less obvious but nevertheless violent ways, enabled the infection and death of many millions.[27]

In the early 1990s, Judith Butler responded to policy decisions by the United States government to divert funds away from research on HIV/AIDS with the critical insight that "'sex' is not only constructed in the service of life or reproduction," as Michel Foucault argued, "but, what might turn out to be a logical corollary, in the service of regulation and apportionment of death."[28] Butler's more nuanced attention to the work of power recognizes that large-scale death continues *through* what Foucault made apparent as the productive or positive work of power with an emphasis on maximizing the biopower of *life*. For not all lives matter in the same way or to the same extent within the emphasis on "life." Reflecting on the HIV/AIDS epidemic, it is immediately apparent—within and between nations—that some lives are made more viable, more endowed, through the unseen or unattended exclusion or refusal of other lives.

As will become increasingly evident, Butler's work plays an important role in this book. In contrast to other modes for deconstructing the self-evidency of distinctions between nature and culture or the biological and social utilized in some sections, Butler's work foregrounds the performative role of intervention that now unwittingly participates in how *only some bodies come to matter*. This is critical in relation to the HIV/AIDS epidemic where, as I have noted, the vast majority of people infected with HIV still do not have access to ARVs. Butler's attention to the political workings of performativity and its generating of the seemingly self-evident or given implicates us *in* the differential nature and effect of interventions. We might ask: How is it that campaigns for vaginal and anal microbicides as alternatives to the problematic gendered reliance on condom use for HIV prevention have only in the last year acquired large scale political, and hence, financial, support when it has been evident from the outset that the male condom is the prerogative of men?[29] How were injecting drug users in Thailand targeted for an HIV biomedical prevention technology trial without the inclusion of free, new needles?[30] Further in reference to the United States, a country where ARVs are long established, how is it that AIDS is the leading cause of death for Black women aged 25–34 years?[31] Questions about the current state of the epidemic abound. When Tony Barnett and Alan Whiteside contend that, "[f]ortunately for humankind, HIV is not a robust virus and it is hard to transmit," they are seeking to draw attention to an epidemic that is enabled by more than a mere biological agent.[32] There is a patterning, or what Butler might term a "performative process," that gives political, ethical, and medical shape to the materiality of the epidemic. As Butler explains of "the real" or, it can be argued, the fleshed outputs of the sense-making of the natural sciences:

> "Materiality" designates a certain effect of power or, rather, is power in its formative or constituting effects. Insofar as power operates successfully by constituting an object domain, a field of intelligibility, as a taken-for-granted ontology, its material effects are taken as material data or primary givens. These material positivities appear outside discourse and power, as incontestable referents, its transcendental signifieds. But this appearance is precisely the moment in which the power/discourse regime is most fully dissimulated and most insidiously effective.[33]

By pursuing Butler's approach to materiality, it becomes possible to open up to question the terrain of HIV objects and subjects, both social and scientific. More specifically, it becomes possible to ask: How can HIV science engage the work of imagination, such that we can devise better interventions? Might a critique of "incontestable referents" enable more innovative thought? More concretely, how does a diagnostic measure function to constitute the person with HIV as a site of surveillance and potential failure?[34] And in what way do the variables of gender, race, and ethnicity found at work in clinical trials reinstate an already presumed organization of bodily difference?[35] As Bruno Latour might argue, interventions, like the matter in which they deal, are already hybrids and generative of further forms of hybridity.[30] Indeed, the potential to generate further forms of hybridity is a central consideration and is reflected in a decision to proceed according to a performative argument—mixing feminist theory and science and technolgy studies—that research, infrastructure, drug therapies, safer sex, and regulation are dynamic entities that acquire their materiality in the course of efforts for more of the same or improvements within.

The phrase "tool box" has frequently been used within the field of cultural studies to convey a mode of inquiry that utilizes different analytic concepts. It is especially apt for describing what follows. In addition to Butler I draw from a range of authors whose work shares an attention to the question of process, that is, to how objects come to acquire their materiality. Indeed, there is no "one size fits all" theoretical approach put forward here. Rather, what I hope to suggest is that a range of analytic tools may be required alongside what is frequently advocated as the need for "a portfolio" of prevention technologies—condoms, drugs, vaccines, microbicides—in the struggle against HIV. In sum, the mix of contributions brought to bear on key areas of concern within the epidemic is intended to contest and reconfigure otherwise seemingly self-evident and, in some instances, intractable features of the epidemic. These contributions overlap but are not demonstrated to cohere into a unified (and hence simplified) theoretical paradigm. Sometimes they are arranged to highlight gaps in the theoretical debate on the question of matter or materiality. At other times, they are used to strengthen and enhance each other.

## CHAPTER OVERVIEW: TRAFFIC, MATERIALITY, AND CONTEMPORARY ISSUES IN ARV-ASSOCIATED HIV

Since much of this book focuses on the effects of ARVs, I begin in chapter 2 with a detailed outline of what are commonly recorded as the unwanted and destructive side effects of ARVs. For some, these effects will be especially familiar. For others for whom this detail is new, it will be clear that despite the advances brought about by ARVs there is still much work to be done. The challenge posed is whether or how critiques of matter, materiality, and "the real" now taking place within feminist theory can provide the HIV field with new modes of engagement. My reference to feminist theory is in direct response to an expression of frustration—and, indeed, some despair—by a renowned scientist on the difficulty of grasping the complexity of the human immune system in the struggle to devise a vaccine for HIV. The nature of his expression—which includes a remark on the place of imagination—serves as a starting point for a conceptual undertaking, in which I use the work of Judith Butler, and its reformulation by Karen Barad, to contest one of the most fundamental presumptions of scientific intervention: namely, the presence of an independent external object or referent that can be objectively deduced, without interference, through the technology that enables it to be known. Although my approach provides a difficult start to the book, insofar as I ask readers to engage with what may seem like abstract philosophical critiques of empiricism, the payoff is that this approach allows me to put in place a series of themes that reoccur throughout the following chapters. I attend to the ways in which the distinction between information and flesh obscures the role of technologies in materializing matter—an issue that raises questions of agency and ethics. This has important implications for understanding how diagnostic tests and drugs partake in the nature of the epidemic. It is intended to suggest to readers both familiar and unfamiliar with HIV biomedicine that a more extensive account of the work of intervention may contribute more directly to what matter might become.

In chapter 3, I approach the critique of matter in terms of what I see as a vacuum in political organizing for better treatment for people living with HIV. Since the emergence of ARVs, forms of activism have been directed toward the urgent need for global access to treatment and—in more local contexts in which such treatments are fully available—toward providing what is termed "treatment information." As a result of these foci of activist efforts, large pharmaceutical companies have, for the most part, acquired the role of determining the substance of what is available for treating. By "substance," I mean pharmaceutical properties, including the devising of certain molecular compounds. Yet, although treatment activism is no longer on the agenda of many nongovernment organizations that now provide highly sophisticated treatment information, the activities of these organizations and their means of dissemination contribute in unrecognized ways to this substance. My aim, then, is to bring this contribution to the foreground and to expose it as a largely untapped resource in a strategy for more "consumer-friendly" ARVs. By recasting the object of consumption as embodying the work of an activity more likely to be identified as occurring at the end stage of pharmaceutical marketing, I propose there is more scope for engagement in, and consequently output of, the pharmaceutical industry. Side-stepping the usual "for-or-against" debates on prescription advertising, my interest is in how texts emerge in this space through the interchange of what Michel Callon and his colleagues term a "hybrid forum"—and how, through the exchanges that make for the hybridity, such texts come to embody a mix of interests.[37] This mix, I argue, marks a potential avenue for more deliberated activity on the part of those who might otherwise understand their relation to "big pharma" as that of a relatively minor actor. Pushing forward the claim of information as flesh, I propose that pharmaceutical substance acquires shape through text. Consequently, the movement and borrowing of text about drugs provides the basis for a renewed form of critique, resonant of pre-ARVs activism, although somewhat different in style.

My argument, in chapter 4, about the need to reconsider modes of intervention is applied to HIV prevention. Although my focus is explicitly on HIV, I begin to make some further links with other areas of biomedical intervention, focusing especially on an area in which biotechnologies are already viewed as generative of behavior. Many people are readily attuned to establishing a causal or at least quasi-causal relationship between the presence of a biotechnological intervention and the practices or behaviors of those for whom biotechnologies have been medically intended. It is not difficult to find examples of this in Western daily media where biomedical advances associated with sex—for instance, the morning-after pill, the vaccine against cervical cancer, or PEP—generate almost knee-jerk queries about "what ill-fated acts will be performed by these potentially irresponsible subjects?" This type of reaction encouraged me to look more closely at the extent to which the causal relation is asserted in relation to sex-associated biomedical phenomena. Sex is therefore an important feature and structuring device in this chapter, all the more so because it has had and continues to have a major role in both transmission and prevention. I begin with a brief review of an earlier period in the HIV epidemic in North America, Western Europe, and Australia and New Zealand, when the practice of sex became an explicit and affirmed theme in prevention education and by way of a celebratory cause in extraordinary forms of political activism. The early period of the epidemic— conventionally marked here as pre-ARVs in contrast to the current context of ARVs—is especially significant because of its emphasis on the role of "the social" as mediating "the biological." Moreover, it can be seen as informing or providing some of the rich informational context that biomedicalization has intensified. This rich informational context is illustrated through interviews with self-identified gay men on negotiating HIV transmission risk.

To respond to the demand for new ways of sustaining HIV prevention and also for dealing with the potentially restrictive moral lens apparent in the case of other biomedical interventions, I recast those targeted by prevention via the notion of "informed matter." I take the phrase from Andrew Barry's work on how the invention of pharmaceutical molecules involves a rich informational context that, ultimately, must come to be embedded in the matter of the molecule.[38] While extrapolating from molecules to gay human subjects may seem a rather big leap, this appropriation of Barry's work is proposed as a step that not only allows us to imagine differently the terrain of prevention, but also to imagine more reflexively the matter or substance of intervention. Rather than simply accept the general presumption of the HIV prevention education field that human practices are informed by knowledge and, therefore, one simply needs more effective knowledge, I draw attention to an historico-material process that—like Barry's molecules—can be seen as embodied in the target. This recasting of the target of prevention provides a subtle but strategic alternative to the more usual viewing of persons as merely acting in response *to*, and subsequent to the event *of*, an intervention. In sum, I argue here that the hybrid forum of prevention messages and biomedicine enacts, in the sense of materializing, increasingly diverse embodied subjects, not simply by means of the deployment of new knowledges of the bodies, but also through its affective—and, hence, ethics-bearing—role in what comes to be lived as the body or condition.

In chapter 5, I shift focus to the "human host" of HIV. This shift follows moves by science—largely driven by the scale of the epidemic and by the evident need for specificity at the level of different individuals—to study human host factors in infection, disease progression, treatment, and biomedical prevention. In practice, molecular genetics as well as epidemiology and behavioral surveillance studies now proceed from the view that the field is constituted according to gender, sex, race, and ethnic differences. In keeping with the critical approach adopted in the preceding chapters, yet at the same time paying more attention to synthesizing some of the divergent approaches employed across these chapters, I examine the way this burgeoning research is becoming enmeshed in the materialization of phenomena that elsewhere is highly contested (especially in other areas of the social sciences and humanities). Despite extensive debates on the sex/gender distinction and on the scientific and political problematics of "race," these categories are being rendered in new ways as a consequence of the goal of achieving better tailored medical interventions. The scope and style of the research is testimony to Paul Rabinow's prediction that molecular genetics will be remade as older cultural categories infuse new ones in ways that, he cautions, will be well worth monitoring.[39] On the one hand, some might wish to shy away from considerations of what are deemed biological differences. This reluctance has obvious historical support, if one considers, for example, the ways that biological explanations have been and continue to be used to support female subordination and the ways that "race" has been used for ideological purposes. On the other hand, the immensely complex field of molecular genetics is rapidly reappropriating everyday conceptions of such differences and returning these as if primary givens.

Bearing in mind Rabinow's caution concerning the ways in which nature and culture may be remade, this penultimate chapter takes up a specific question: How is it possible to talk about difference in ways that enliven scientific debates and vivify intervention, without falling back into the logic of differentially designated notions of difference? I draw on contributions from those who engage questions of gender, sex, and race in both feminist theory and science and technology studies. I am especially interested in the extent to which it may be helpful to think about the representation of human host difference(s) as the performative effect of scientific methodologies. And, further, how the performative account might be developed by incorporating materiality as a dynamic affected by but also affecting intervention. Consistent with the overall aim of this book, this chapter poses an array of issues that do not simply confound the information/flesh distinction but, in addition, suggest the need for a more historically specific relational conception of matter as the basis for intervention.

While this book primarily aims to develop new modes of thinking about—and intervening in—the course of HIV/AIDS, its capacity to do so will be at least partially dependent on how effectively it draws from the contribution of pre-ARV cultural interventions. As I indicated earlier, the work that has already gone into contesting the relationship between information and flesh and the inventive way that information—in the form of prevention education—has altered HIV is especially important. I refer here to the use, for example, of condoms and prevention education to affect and reduce the movement of the virus across bodies. From this perspective, it is possible to say that a borrowing or traffic between information and flesh has long formed part of the strategic response to HIV transmission. Even so, this style of engagement—premised largely on HIV as culturally affected, as if prevention can continue by putting aside a more intensified and productive medical presence—is no longer adequate.

With tragic irony, it is the most mundane and ordinary of infections that underscore the urgent need to query current strategies and, moreover, the importance of examining the relational work of information and flesh. Candida albicans, more readily known as oral thrush (a white furry fungus in the throat), is a frequent and seemingly inconsequential form of opportunistic infection that falls under the umbrella term of AIDS. Although readily treatable with "over-the-counter drugs," oral thrush is a killer for those without the money to purchase these drugs when marketed at inhibitively high prices in developing countries. People in these countries can die from severe thrush because it makes it impossible to eat or drink.[40] While the sort of work I undertake here in response to molecular-oriented treatments has little direct bearing on this phenomenon of thrush-induced deaths, the example of no treatment most potently emphasizes the stakes in examining the relationality of information and flesh. How can we know of such deaths? By what means is it possible to discern that these happen, despite the means for prevention? Is the act of observation ethically implicated?[41] Or, through what dynamic of complex relations are bodies made available to yield this information? Questions such as these are all too easy to pose in the context of an epidemic that, according to the range of international sponsor, advocacy, and normative agencies that address HIV/AIDS, spans the extremes of poverty and sophisticated molecular knowledge. HIV infection is only bracketed off from AIDS for some people and in intensely complex ways. As I have already noted, my intention is to examine more closely where and in what ways the concepts of information and flesh are mobilized by focusing on the associative work of biomedical advance. While I see biomedicine as a vast area of gain, it is not sufficiently so that it warrants uncritical acceptance and expansion. As the effort to deal with the epidemic is extraordinarily insufficient in terms of drugs and diagnostic provision, even basic primary care, I argue here it is also conceptually insufficient to its perceived challenges.

My title, *HIV Interventions: Biomedicine and the Traffic between Information and Flesh*, is a reminder that there is something slippery in the matter of our thinking. That is to say, thinking and the means by which it takes place are difficult to hold apart; indeed, the very suggestion that one is attempting to do so could be seen as an oxymoron. Nevertheless, it is still necessary to engage the distinction in order to proceed with intervention. And, more so, to recognize that intervention is more effective, more productive, more generative—although not necessarily in desired or welcomed ways—than when conceived according to the traditions of classical realism in post-Enlightenment science, tackled throughout. Traffic recognizes a movement between entities of difference—although it may be a movement that helps constitute their difference as much as dissolve it.

# 2

## IMAGINATION, DIAGNOSTICS, AND
## THE MATERIALIZATION OF HIV

Imagination: The action of imagining or forming mental images or concepts of external objects not present to the senses; the result of this process.
The mental faculty which forms images or concepts of external objects not
present to the senses, and of their relations (to each other or to the subject).
Scheming or devising; a devise, a plan, a plot; a fanciful project. Expectation,
anticipation. The faculty of fanciful thought; fancy. The creative faculty of the
mind; the ability to frame new and striking concepts. The mind; thinking;
thought, opinion.

—The New Shorter Oxford English Dictionary

WITHIN THE HIV FIELD, IT IS NOW WELL ESTABLISHED THAT A VARIED
and complex array of unwanted effects accompany the achievement
of ARVs. Some of these so deemed "side" effects are known to be potentially lethal. They include heart disease, liver damage, diabetes, hyperten-
sion, nerve damage (peripheral neuropathy), pancreatitis, and bone diseases
(osteoporosis, osteonecrosis). Others, namely lipodystrophy (fat redistribu-
tion that forms a "buffalo hump" on the upper back below the neck, expands
the torso, especially around the waist, and causes significantly enlarged
breasts in women) and lipoatrophy (fat loss most visible on the arms, legs,
face, and buttocks) are distressingly disfiguring, if not disabling. In addition
to these unwanted effects there are the more mundane ones that affect day-
to-day life and that, for some sufferers, are highly distressing and disruptive
even if not regarded as medically serious, such as insomnia, nightmares,
depression, chronic diarrhea, nausea, vomiting, and stomach cramps.[1]
Added to these side effects is the almost unmanageable nature of some dos-

ing regimens that can require taking up to seven pills three times a day and at different specified periods, before food, with food, and after food. "Poor adherence" to difficult dosing regimens is often held responsible for insufficient drug absorption, which is understood, in turn, to enable strains of the virus to replicate and mutate.[2] Indeed, concern about the relationship between adherence and the management of viral replication and mutation, which I expand on below, is so significant within the HIV field that it serves as a recurring theme throughout this book.

Not surprisingly, the highly toxic nature of the drug therapies and the likelihood that the virus will become resistant to the drugs are both features in clinical decision making, in the design of HIV behavioral surveillance and prevention, and in ongoing biomedical intervention research. Everyday HIV medical consultations involve complicated and uncertain decisions along the lines of when to commence combination therapy, given the damaging effects of the drugs, and what combination of drugs should be used, given the difficulty of adhering to strict dosing regimes. As one clinician stated in reference to the changes brought to the clinic with the advent of antiretrovirals:[3]

> Pre-1996 my clinics were full of people who I would see every month or every few weeks and manage their symptoms. . . , progressive immuno-deficiency, gradually more disabled. . . , then come into hospital and die. . . . That's now changed completely. I now maybe only have a few people who have severe immuno-deficiency, where we're having problems in treating their HIV infection because of multi-drug resistance. My clinics are now largely to do with therapy, managing the response to therapy, managing the side effects of therapy, monitoring HIV infection in those people not on therapy and it's become very much chronic disease management, definitely.

The quote offers insight into the way that HIV has been transformed by ARVs in the space of the clinic but, more important for what I cover in this chapter, it highlights how this space has become technologized through new knowledges and instruments. Further, with these have come new phenomena mostly articulated through reference to drug resistance and drug side effects. In what follows, I use the problem of side effects and drug resistance as a provocation to contest the self-evidence of the framework from which side effects and drug resistance arise. My focus is directed to the work of technologies in materializing these challenges. My aim is to inquire into the distinction between information and flesh on which scientific work proceeds and, in doing so, foreground the possibility for rethinking the HIV terrain. The basis for this rethinking draws on recent critiques of matter in feminist theory, used here to highlight how science is ethically implicated in what would more usually be presumed as its objects *for* intervention. That is to say, this chapter proceeds by contesting one of the most fundamental presumptions of scientific intervention, the presence of an independent external object or referent that can be objectively deduced without interference of the technology that enables it to be known. In place of the seemingly necessary presumption of an objectively knowable object, a more extensive account of scientific work and, hence inventiveness, is proposed as not only possible but already available in its process.

To undertake this task I utilize a performative account of matter that may be contrasted with the realism of HIV science. To elaborate this, I want to briefly switch back to the empirical of the science of HIV and why I have introduced this chapter with a definition of imagination. For the notion of imagination serves as an important linking device for bringing critiques of matter into dialogue with HIV science. In reference to a discussion about the difficulty of developing a vaccine to prevent and possibly treat HIV, Joseph McCune, a highly reputed HIV scientist, states that the human immune system is so complex that it "hinders the discovery and development of effective vaccines and therapies." Following on from this observation, McCune provides the addendum, as a consequence "much remains left to the imagination."[4] Although the statement is unlikely to have been made with any reference to epistemological and ontological debates now taking place regarding performative accounts of matter—notably in what I refer to as poststructural feminist theory or to those in science and technology studies (STS)—I will use it as license to propose that imagination may be more pervasive and, therefore, more significant to HIV interventions than McCune recognizes.

I deduce from McCune's claim that in the absence of "real" knowledge of bodily matter and virus, imagination is seen as outside real knowledge. Although, it is important to add, this does not necessarily deny its contribution. Indeed, according to McCune, it seems the contrary is so. And, for this reason, I retain an idea of its contributory function throughout the chapter.

What struck me when I first came across the distinction between real or, as McCune might himself say, empirically tested evidence in contrast to more fanciful thought on the constitutive nature of "the real" was its juxtaposition with the critique of matter provided by Butler and the reformulation of this by Karen Barad. Recent debate within this area of feminist theory provides an almost perverse counter to McCune and to the style of thought expressed. Rather than considering imagination as an activity outside or external to the real, the work of Butler and Barad can be read to suggest that imagination—as a mode of thought contrary to the presumptions of objective scientific knowledge—is always present and inherent to what we take to be an external, unmediated "real."

While HIV may be conceived by science as an object qualified only by the inadequacy of knowledge, its ontological status must inevitably be in dispute or, at least, conditional for a substantial part of the field of poststructuralist feminism. In the course of this chapter, I want to use these differing positions of science and feminist poststructuralist critique to challenge and extend each other. For while there is clear evidence that science is limited in its grasp of HIV, there is much debate within social theories of matter that may help to explain at least some of why this is so. In the early sections of this chapter, I outline some of the key premises of Butler's theory of performativity for illuminating a *process* by which material entities come to *appear* as given. I then move to its reformulation by Barad for addressing a more science studies set of concerns, prior to directing these contributions to the matter of HIV.

## LOCATING "THE BIOLOGICAL"

Butler begins her book *Bodies That Matter*: "Is there a way to link the question of the materiality of the body to the performativity of gender?"[5] Performativity, she explains, "must be understood not as a singular or deliberate 'act,' but, rather, as the reiterative and citational practice by which discourse produces the effects that it names."[6] Reiteration is imperative because "materialization is never quite complete, . . . bodies never quite comply with the norms by which their materialization is impelled."[7] To put it another way, the material or real world is imagined in the sense that we come to know it through reiterative practices that are, in themselves, normative.[8] For instance, the performative of gender—which materializes sex difference—begins for Butler at the moment of our birth with the imperative of the speech act, "it's a girl" or "it's a boy."[9] Despite evidence to show that bodies do not always conform to the binary of male or female—through intersexed or indeterminate sex organs and varying reproductive capacity—the binary continues to be accepted as a reference *to* a self-evident biological fact.[10] This self-evidency is the consequence of a process of gendering and so extensive that, even when medical "correction" becomes part of the performative, the investment in the binary as "given" continues unquestioned.[11] The normative or what Butler terms the process of "investiture" is, then, that which makes the intelligible as such and, most importantly, involves what she later points to as a process sustained through exclusion.[12]

Butler's emphasis on investiture, or what might be termed the deployment of the regulatory ideal or norm, distinguishes her notion of performativity from other uses of the term, for instance by STS scholars such as Bruno Latour, John Law, and Michel Callon, whose work I shall also engage in the course of this book. Indeed, the emphasis on investiture will be recalled in conjunction with or alongside such other contributors when discussing the process of materialization in later chapters. I have elected to begin with Butler's approach because it provides a critical handle on not only how the distinction between "information" and "flesh" or the "biological" and "cultural" might be challenged. It also provides a basis for why this may be important. That is to say, at its core, Butler's use of performativity is a political endeavor intended to reveal the way in which materialization takes place in interested ways—although not in a humanist but, rather, historical sense.[13]

However, it needs to be said that translating Butler's performative into the field of science is no straightforward or entirely satisfactory matter. For other than an attention to the materialization of sexed bodies, her work does not specifically deal with the performative work of science. By concentrating on the question of how power works *through* ontological claims, Butler's work will be shown as valuable to a highly nuanced query of the powers of imaginative work but not especially helpful on the question of how an alternative ontology might be formulated. In short, her notion of the coextensive nature of materiality and investiture—whereby materiality is always an effect of its coextensive relation with technologies of knowledge—is both enabling and disenabling. For some it aligns her with the problematic approach of social construction-ism that—in its privileging of a notion of culture or discourse, especially in reference to the body—can be argued to lose sight of what is at stake in performing this position.[14] Although Butler claims that materiality is not *only* investiture: "nature has a history, and not merely a social one," it is difficult to see how she might account for nature's history that moves beyond a culturalist conception.[15] Consequently, it is difficult to use her argument to elicit the contributory presence of matter in its own materialization.

According to Vicki Kirby, an erasure takes place when we distinguish culture from nature and, specifically, in the assigning of language as the property of culture (and not also nature).[16] The very features that are ascribed to culture—literacy and numeracy—can be observed in nature, for example, in the work of DNA. As Kirby says: "it [nature] is already a writing system whose re-presentation of itself disrupts the purity and integrity imputed to it."[17] Provocatively, Kirby suggests a new ethical field whereby "scientists might have to question the implicit humanism of their practice and consider that perhaps the objects that have *drawn* their attention are, in fact, attracting that intention, subjecting themselves to mutual inspection and reflexive involvement."[18] Importantly, although the argument is centered on scientific understanding, it is intended as a challenge to those social constructionists who have become preoccupied with language in what can be characterized as a somewhat reductive, exclusionary manner. Kirby highlights how social constructionist argu-ments assume and, moreover, reify a problematic notion of "culture." This emphasis on "culture" prevents a more cogent response to a world where flesh is ever-present. For, ironically, it desists from engagement with what Butler might say matters. In Kirby's view, the over attach-ment to "culture" as if wholly distinct from nature means that "[mat-ter's] palpability and its physical insistence, is rendered unspeakable and unthinkable."[19] As a consequence, we have little purchase on what takes place, for example, in the everyday mundane of the workplace or the possibly exotic of the laboratory. As a growing number in this field of study have done, Kirby points to the need for a methodological approach able to provide insight into the materialization of phenomena not already designated as information *or* flesh.[20]

Hence, while on the one hand Butler will be demonstrated here to offer an important basis from which to devise methodological innovation, her performative account requires some additional work to enjoin it to the physical insistence found in HIV diagnostics and treatment. The challenge, yet also what I shall argue is of key import in her work, lies in the way the object of science is contested. For on the basis that bodies and other biological matter emerge through, rather than prior to, reiterative processes, Butler's performativity can be said to dispense with the notion of a referent. Or more precisely, as Mariam Fraser puts this, we are offered "a theory of political transformation informed by, and dependent upon, the inability of (human) language to capture the material referent."[21] It is, therefore, a theory that refutes the possibility of neutral/objective knowing in a very immediate sense. For such knowing assumes a process without political effect, as claimed by the natural sciences. This departure from objective knowing—in the sense of the natural sciences—has significant implications for the question of intervention. "Objects" as effects of knowledge are open to question for the manner in which they have come to acquire their apparency. But, in turn, it is necessary to ask: If "the referent" cannot be captured, how can intervention proceed? Or, similarly, how can the contributing work of non-discursive matter be approached?

According with the general tone of this book and the impetus to pursue a critique of science, in part, along the lines presented by Butler's theory of performativity and Kirby's incisive contribution, an optimistic view would suggest that among the many possibilities available through the interrogation of all "givens" and, linked to this, a refuting of claims of objectivity, is an extension or opening up of the very notion of what social, political, and/or ethical intervention might involve. In the context of this chapter, this position will be developed as the basis for reviewing the emergence of "the body," "the virus," "drugs," and "person with HIV" in HIV biomedicine. The impossibility of achieving a transparent *re-presentation* of the objects of HIV, human immune systems, and drug therapies—as if unaffected by technologies involved in their representation—will provide ground for what I hope is a robust challenge to science. Robust in the sense of what it might enable in the future development of interventions, now called upon by McCune to require imagination. To put it another way, I consider how the instability of material-semiotic empirically grounded objects—as set out by science—may be important to dealing with the challenge of HIV.[22] Specifically, I propose that this instability may enable HIV medical science to reflect on its already active imaginative role in materializing HIV. Further, I shall propose that the dilemma of having no referent may be replaced by a contingent *quasi*-referent that is not outside language or other forms of technology but, rather, *of* them.

## THE APPEARANCE OF PHENOMENA

In her essay "Getting Real: Technoscientific Practices and the Materialization of Reality," Barad extends Butler's performativity beyond the reiteration of utterances in the materializing of objects.[23] Barad's expressed intention is to provide new conceptual tools to enable Butler's theory of performativity to recognize the contributory role of more than language (in the discursive sense) in the materialization of matter. To undertake this reformulation of Butler, Barad focuses on the ultrasound machine and the manner in which it materializes or achieves what comes to be known as a fetus. Her analysis draws attention to the relationship or, as she puts this, intra-activity of machine, discourse, and human body matter. Retaining Butler's feminist endeavor that attends to the way bodies come to matter, Barad provides a critique of the process of materialization that reveals the work of a prior liberal or neo-liberal discourse in giving form to the fetus and, at the same time, shows how this is co-constitutive with its targeted matter. The fetus of ultrasound technology is enacted through the movement of sound waves that—in their design—enlist matter to materialize a seemingly free-floating fetus, wholly independent of the maternal body. In effect, the fetus appears as a precursor to liberal personhood in possession of inalienable rights and, thus, available to anti-abortion discourse that asserts fetal rights in contradistinction to those of the mother.

Apparent from Barad's analysis is a process of materialization that involves a discursively shaped technology engaging bodily matter in biotechnologically effected, inclusive and exclusive ways. Hence, while the ultrasound machine is understood within the diagnostic field as an apparatus *for* observation, its design or the nature of its operation comes to be embedded in what is, otherwise, presumed as simply observed. "The fetus" performed by ultrasound technology is not an object in the terms assumed by the natural sciences. It is, in the phrasing of Barad, a "phenomenon" in the sense that it stands as objectively knowable because of the intra-active process through which it has been materialized. Its form is contingent on the type of apparatus used in its materialization and, importantly, an apparatus in which human agency has a role.

By filling the space of intelligibility previously occupied by the referent, the notion of phenomenon provides the possibility for a recasting of empirical matter that acknowledges the conditions of its realness. The notion of phenomenon exposes medical science as invariably co-implicated in the objects that it presumes to be available as objectively true.[24] This relation is named "agential realism" by Barad in order to underscore the presence of human agency in what is assumed as "the real." Similar to "intra-activity," the term "agential realism" foregrounds an activity different to that usually presumed, for it recognizes the mix of the conceptual in technological design and effect plus the matter subject to such design.[25] In part, "agential realism" might be regarded as analogous to what Butler deems the work of "investiture" and the insidious way this style of power conceals its operations in a mythical real, that is, in a real that appears as if prior to and distinct from that which it is assumed to merely speak *of*.[26] But it is also an attempt to allow for a more material performativity with emphasis on the role of the non-discursive, namely the eliciting of human substance by biomedical technologies. Indeed, in its reformulation of performativity to allow for a more satisfactory recognition of the co-constitutive role of investiture and materiality, the emphasis on human agency sets it apart from STS approaches taken up later in this book. It is clear that for Barad, human agency is ethically accountable for the material conditions of the world in ways that other "non-human" actors or contributors are not.[27] As she puts this: "we are not only responsible for the knowledge that we seek but, in part, for what exists."[28] This process, whereby flesh is elicited through the technologies of human design and therefore materialized through human sense-making, means that we as "human" are directly implicated in what comes to be received and acted on as if objectively real. Barad characterizes this as an "apparatus" that is ongoing and transformative. It not only reflects what has gone into its capacities but, with these capacities, engenders new and ongoing dynamics. Consequently, we can be held in some way responsible for the materialization of phenomena because, as she explains, "it is sedimented out of particular practices that we have a role in shaping."[29]

> Apparatuses are not pre-existing or fixed entities; they are themselves constituted through particular practices that are perpetually open to rearrangements, rearticulations, and other reworkings. . . . Furthermore, any particular apparatus is always in the process of intra-acting with other apparatuses, and the enfolding of phenomena (which may be traded across space, time, and subcultures only to find themselves differently materializing) into subsequent iterations of particular situated practices . . . that result in the production of new phenomena, and so on.[30]

Since this is a deliberately different conception of agency and of bioethics than usually found in biomedicine and in debates on the nature of consent and responsibility, it poses a challenge to how we conceive of materiality and, moreover, to how we conceive our role in what appears as materiality. At its core, Barad's argument echoes Butler's in that objects are already imbued with imagination through our interventions—scientific, social scientific, and more—and at least one task in the achievement of better HIV science may be to incorporate this within the field of vision. Or, on the basis of Butler's claim, "there is no reference to a pure body which is not at the same time a further formation of that body,"[31] it is critical that we pay heed to the generative work of our interventions. In specific reference to the use of diagnostics in association with ARVs, the process of formation may be regarded as critical. The unintended and unwanted phenomena mentioned earlier suggest that these technologies are formative and in ways that warrant not necessarily *more* imagination but, rather, a mode of examination that is attentive to this already generative feature of their work.

## THE VIRAL LOAD TEST, MATERIALIZING HIV

While the medical field might more usually be viewed as comprised of a series of distinct objects with fixed properties measurable by transparent means, Barad's work makes possible a recasting of these as an array of phenomena, the properties of which are constituted, in part, by a prior imagining. Following the example of ultrasound technology, the current materialization of HIV can be traced to a series of medical technologies that are shaped by and shaping of phenomena otherwise understood as objectively and impartially imaged.[32] Here, I concentrate on the pivotal HIV biotechnology commonly referred to as the viral load test and examine its role in materializing the substance of HIV, the embodied subject with HIV, and drug-resistant HIV as part of an ongoing dynamic.

Although what I present below goes some way toward a reconceived notion of the ontology of HIV and other seemingly distinct objects associated with it, the argument that I put forward is not inconsistent with the way that HIV science has, according to its own trajectory, conceived and then reconceived the nature of HIV. Where my approach significantly diverges is in its attention to the processes that enact the virus. Like the fetus, the virus, as it appears, is an approximation achieved through highly sophisticated but nevertheless selective and, as will also be apparent, reiterative practices. In the remainder of this chapter it should become apparent that there is no stable object that we refer to as "HIV" or "the virus." On the one hand, it is revealed by science as having altered over the course of the epidemic as a consequence of its movement and mixing with bodies and now, especially, with ARVs and associated observational technologies. On the other hand, though, there is a certain abstracting out of what is involved in this mixing—on the part of science—in order to achieve a seemingly stable object *of* study *for* intervention.

These dual aspects of scientific engagement with HIV are evident in the way HIV has changed as an object within the laboratory and clinical medicine. Familiar to those in the HIV field, will be the way that the virus came into view in the very early 1980s through tests for detecting antibodies that continue to be read as a sign of viral presence.[33] The absence of visible disease symptoms, but indication of present antibodies, contributed to an accepted hypothesis that the virus remained in a latent, that is, non-destructive state in vivo and for some years prior to the onset of AIDS.[34] In terms of my argument, it is possible to say that the virus as it is currently understood had not materialized in vivo. For if the virus is no longer believed by credible scientists to have a latent phase—as it was conceived—and although there are debates about when to start taking ARVs, there is acceptance across the scientific field that the presumption of a latent phase slowed research into how to use the drugs most effectively.[35]

In the mid-90s, the advent of the viral load test, able to measure viral particles, materialized HIV in a different way and paved the way for new understandings of viral replication.[36] Increased knowledge of the ways through which the virus is able to enter human cells and co-opt the workings of these cells meant that the use of antiretroviral drugs was rethought and monotherapy (one antiretroviral drug) was replaced by combination therapy or treatment (usually a combination of two or three antiretrovirals). Now the viral load test is regularly carried out on an HIV (antibody) positive individual's sample of peripheral blood to provide surrogate markers of disease progression in the form of measures of viral particles, weighed along with CD4 cell counts (measure of immune cells). If the viral particle count is determined as "high" and the CD4 cell count as "low" then ARVs may be introduced.[37] If the person is on ARVs, increases in the number of viral particles over time may serve as an indicator that the virus is becoming resistant to the drugs.

Drug resistance is a phenomenon linked in much prevalent scientific thinking—although not all, as I go on to discuss—to the sustaining of consistent drug levels in vivo and presumed to be prevented or significantly so through near perfect dosing adherence. Failure to sustain adequate drug levels is believed to allow the virus to not just replicate but to favor replication of mutated virus insensitive to the drugs present. The emergence of drug sensitive virus is of immediate concern because it may reduce an individual's existing drug options, compounding the tricky negotiation of side effects that most usually require a broad range of drug options.[38] Less immediate, but nevertheless worrying, the emergence of drug insensitive virus poses a threat to the current reliance on drugs for managing existing infection within a population. Hence, even before an individual begins taking ARVs, assessment may be made of his/her capacity to take all the pills in a combination therapy and at the correct times.[39] Some clinicians may consider whether their patient's lifestyle is conducive to regular or "near perfect" dosing, especially if the person is leading what is sometimes termed a "chaotic" lifestyle.[40]

Until recently, pill-taking or, more usually termed, dosing has been regarded as a fairly onerous task. There are many studies that show that remembering to take the pills at set times; fitting this into a public schedule without having to disclose the reason for dosing; and/or the difficulty of swallowing pills, even to the point of gagging or vomiting, is not easy or straightforward for many.[41] Without disregarding the apparent paramount importance of dosing, it is possible to see that the viral load test is involved in a performative of the ideal/normative patient who is constituted through the presumptions of dosing and, as Kane Race points out, the linking of "matters of sex and infectivity, lifestyle and medication consumption, and prognosis."[42] Although the viral load test may be lauded for the gains that ARVs are able to perform against viral replication, Race shows how the test has engendered HIV in new ways. HIV is still present but made invisible at the community level, to become a privatized individual matter and a matter where more specific assessments of infectivity are probable (discussed in chapter 4), where dosing is part of everyday life (discussed in chapter 3), and whereby the day-to-day experience involves, as Race puts this, a "process of constant monitoring and vigilance around the presence of the Other (the virus)."[43] The optimal test result of "undetectable" does not free the individual from HIV. Rather, in freeing up the subject from the status of abject/infectious, Race explains, "it also implants an imperative around the individual self-surveillance upon which the subject's capacity to retain (non-contaminate) status depends."[44]

Continuing on from the incisive way Race presents the work of the viral load test, it is apparent that underpinning the imperative of retaining "undetectable" or consistent viral load status are the presumptions that dosing is achievable through embodied will and that it results in viral suppression.[45] But the link between dosing, self will, near perfect adherence, and "undetectable" or consistent viral load are not always borne out. For instance, there is now data that indicates that missing pills does not necessarily result in a significant increase to viral load. There is also data indicating that viral resistance can occur in the context of "good" adherence.[46] Moreover, in some of the scientific literature viral resistance is attributed to other complex and likely interrelated causal factors. These include possible different drug absorption rates in individuals and/or the presence of other drugs, dietary conditions, extra vitamin intakes, or genetics.[47] Indeed, the very notion of "resistance" has been argued as misleading. According to Jonathan Schapiro, an unwitting conflation takes place in the metaphor and the grounds on which it is used:

Our ability to quantify resistance in such terms as "fold increase" [a type of measurement] may satisfy our desire for quantification; however, at the same time, it encourages our belief that this information alone provides an answer to our questions. Such answers are not definitive; the virus does not know that we call it "resistant" when a susceptibility assay records a certain-fold increase in IC [inhibitory concentration of a drug].[48]

On the basis of the above, we might read the facts of "resistance" as evidence of the variability of HIV as a force and the failure to register this variability or heterogeneity as another more insidious exclusion in the constituting of the embodied subject, responsible for his or her viral load levels *and*, moreover, the virus itself. But besides this attention to the materialization of a potential non-adherent subject and delimited virus, variability in HIV can be conceived as part of a more ongoing transformative dynamic illustrated through the emergent properties of "resistant" and "wild type" virus. While mutations or "resistant virus" are materialized as such in the presence of ARVs, there is also the variability that may become evident with the withdrawal of ARVs. "Wild type" is a term used to characterize a strain of virus apart from drug effects, either before or after withdrawal from drug therapies.[49] It can be a form more virulent as well as drug sensitive. For those struggling with how to respond to the development of viral resistance, the variability of "fitness" or viability for replication and destruction can be weighed against drug-resistant mutations "whose infectivity, replication, or protein maturation . . . is impaired."[50] In other words, the variability between "wild type" and a less "fit" drug-resistant form gives rise to a debate over whether to continue or cease therapies in the presence of drug resistance.[51] From a Barad perspective, the materialization of viral variability could be argued as enabled by the viral load test in at least two ways: the viral load test is part of the knowledge (and network) construction of drug interventions; and, through viral load readings, the drug therapies are used with the effect of changing what is observed (materialized) as a materially altered virus.[52]

## THE PALPABLE PRESENCE OF HIV, DRUGS, AND BODY MATTER

Drug resistant and "wild type" viruses occur because, according to scientific accounts, the human immunodeficiency virus exists, as I have already noted, through replication and, with this, mutation. In other words, it seems the virus is never stable. Yet, perversely, the concept of instability or, more appropriately enduring but changing, appears to be a difficult one to grasp. Or, perhaps more precisely, it is difficult to imagine within a linear cause/effect and subject/object framing as this framing involves a series of normative and exclusionary measures. Drugs do not always result in viral suppression. Nor do they, directly, produce viral resistance. And, while dosing contributes to changes in the virus, the changes are not reducible to an act of self-will over or external to the virus. The conceptualizing of what an enduring and transformative virus involves is already delimited by the presumption of an object that can be observed and extracted as distinct from that involved in its materiality. Even the lay person, familiar with HIV medical science, is aware of how the viral load test is subject to temporal and spatial inclusions and exclusions. Viral load tests must be repeated at regular intervals because results change. They are carried out in peripheral blood and the results must then be extrapolated, without certainty, to other locales in the body also subject to viral activity and damage.[53] Linked to these qualifiers is the question of what "undetectable" means for infectivity, for instance: Does "undetectable" mean nil or insignificant risk of transmission? (In chapter 4 this possibility is shown to be a relational factor in the shift of current sexual practice among gay communities).[54] Further, factors such as the presence of other infections and/or genetic differences are believed to affect viral capacities, that is, in the presence of another sexually transmitted infection the effects of the virus may differ.[55]

The properties identified as those of the virus are already recognized, within science, as provisional. But not in a manner that includes the extensive contributory work of diagnostic methods. The latter may be recognized as unable to provide full knowledge of the virus and even though different test sensitivity is known to affect the viral load measure, the role of diagnostic methods in giving shape to what is seen remains qualified and contained. Hence the object of virus continues to be presumed as transparently knowable and represented, despite the scientific evidence to show otherwise. The presumption follows from the classical realist conception of scientific work *discovering* what is already there or bringing together elements of what is already there to achieve a new effect. Important to stress at this point is that to recognize that HIV is a phenomenon affected by the process of its identification does not take away from its palpable presence, its insistence as a force to be contested. Nor does this recognition take away from the ability of medical science to intervene—although not as directly or neatly as it may be anticipated —in the biological substance of its imaginary. But it does highlight the performative nature of science and how science achieves more than is usually assumed. To put it another way, a performative account of the materialization of matter makes apparent the contributory work of science *in* the substance of its study.

By providing tools to enable a more self-reflexive critique of medical science, Butler and Barad's theory of performativity allows critical reflection on the role of imagination at the very point where science and its object are presumed distinct. This recasting, to consider the pre-existent presence of imagination, contests the self-evidency of the difficulties as they are framed within HIV medical science. It therefore opens up the field to more and different ways of considering these difficulties, even a reframing of the nature of the difficulty. In doing so, it also recasts the debate on matter. The potential of a poststructuralist critique called into question on the grounds that it is unable to sufficiently or adequately engage with the substance of the non-discursive, may be rethought in light of the variability of HIV. In the absence of a fixed entity and, in its place, the emergence of a series of changing associations suggests that what is required is not only an account of palpability or intra-activity but a processual one. The matter of HIV—like other mixings of matter—is a provocation to devise a performative account attentive to the more dynamic and therefore ongoing formative nature of materialization.

## CONCLUSION

Although the question of the referent provided the starting point for this chapter and whether or how it is possible to intervene in the epidemic if the object cannot be presumed to be unaffected by technologies of knowledge and hardware, the nature of HIV—if we are to follow the empirical of science—suggests the question is redundant. The science inferred conception of a prior entity that is sufficiently stable or self-identical that it can be tracked, measured, and acted *upon* without having already been affected, is revealed by the empirical matter of science as a fallacy. Observational technologies such as the viral load test are active in the materialization of the object, *imagined* as external to the observational process. Further, in their materializing of the substance of HIV, they are productive of other or new forms of matter. The unwanted exemplars of the viral load test are resistant and wild-type virus, two forms of viruses that have materialized with the viral load test in association with ARVs.

In other words, imagination—defined in the opening to this chapter as "fanciful thought" or "the ability to frame new and striking concepts"—is not outside the performative process. This challenge to McCune's assumption that the achievements of science may require imagination, suggests that science already has much at hand. Further, since imagining cannot be separated out from intervention, it is imperative that novel ways of working with and through it are devised. This follows from Butler's argument that the performative process is an operation that must take place because bodies do not, "in fact," accord materially with their normative investiture. The theory of performativity outlined above gives emphasis to the need for an extended or, more specifically, reflexive scientific imagining. While the palpable presence of matter continues to elude the realist grasp, according to the Butler/Barad performative, its palpability is apparent in the need for reiterative citation. If this is so, as I have argued above, and the reiteration can be witnessed in a performative of "resistant" and "wild-type" virus then these entities might be revised. Paradoxically, they are performatively presumed and enacted by intervention as enduring while also evidenced as altering in their relations with not just ARVs and a host of other spatial and temporally presumed phenomena. Viral resistance and reversion to "wild type" demonstrate that matter—as science might claim it—is not, in itself, inert but, rather, insistent in ways that have and will continue to be invested by the processes of observation and other intervention, namely pharmaceutical.

In many respects as I have indicated, the contingent nature of the virus is already well known to science. It will come as no surprise to most HIV specialist clinicians and scientists that the viral load test results need to be assessed with reference to the sensitivity of the test, the presence or absence of ARVs, and the possible co-factors affecting viral resistance. But the characterizing of scientific intervention as a form of agential realism, whereby science is ethically implicated in its otherwise seemingly "given" objects, may present a new series of challenges and especially as it calls upon science to recognize an already imagination-imbued work. In methodological terms this may mean a more extensive reckoning with the generative nature of seemingly objective instruments, such as the viral load test in its production of surrogate markers or of ARVs in their design of viral resistance.

# 3

# HIV: A SYNERGY OF BIOLOGICAL MATTER, BIOTECHNOLOGICAL MATTER, AND PUBLICS

Language itself is "real" and "material," a concrete vehicle that lays a trail of its existence in documents, policies, conversations, and other sites and routes of cultural circulation.

—Paula A. Treichler, *How to Have Theory in an Epidemic:*
*Cultural Chronicles of AIDS*

TAKING A LEAD FROM TREICHLER'S STATEMENT ABOVE AND, FURTHER, her claim that "ultimately, the activities and ideas that we organize around the sign AIDS—including the chronicles that we write—have the power to change the fate of the epidemic," I want to consider the potential of text to inform the substance of drugs.[1] Treichler's emphasis on the significance of language was developed pre-HIV antiretroviral combination therapies. If she did foresee, at the time, that a major turn would occur in the epidemic with the development of ARVs, she may not have considered taking on the political force of multinational drug manufacturers, or big pharma as they are often called, for the problems with ARVs. Using language (in the more limited linguistic and not anthropological sense)[2] as a lobbying tactic to challenge homophobia and to gain political support for treatments may be regarded as different from intervening in the pharmaceutical design of treatments. That is to say, lobbying *for* drugs is different from lobbying for improvements *in* drugs. Nevertheless, and moving on from the critique of matter that I began in the previous chapter, Treichler's claim provides a valuable point of orientation for a new lobbying tactic intended to improve drug substance.

My hypothesis is that some traction in the struggle for better biomedical interventions can be gained through consideration of the coextensive or co-constitutive relation of sign or linguistic text and pharmaceutical compound. To "test" and, in doing so, "demonstrate" the validity for such a hypothesis, I proceed by mapping some of the textual exchanges that inform the development of one particular ARV combination therapy called Trizivir, manufactured by the multinational corporation GlaxoSmithKline.[3] The exchanges that I foreground will be understood according to what Michel Callon and his colleagues have characterized as a "hybrid forum," which captures a dynamic interplay of various actors—ranging from scientists and corporations to patient activists—coming together to affect market outcomes through reflexive engagement with each other. As Callon and his colleagues put this, different actors question aspects of the market and "based on an analysis of . . . [market] functioning, try to conceive and establish new rules for the game."[4] Although Callon and his colleagues do not refer to the field of HIV drug development, their concept of an interplay of diverse actors has immediate resonance. The notion of a "hybrid forum" can be understood as an historical development in Patton's account of an earlier period of HIV treatment activism:

> By about 1987, anarchic protests known as "treatment activism" had forced
> a new understanding of people who had contracted HIV: They had become
> active participants—consumers of medical care—rather than passive victims.
> By hammering away at soft points in scientific nomenclature, drug market-
> ing, and ethical frameworks, this form of activism helped prompt researchers
> and ethics boards in the United States to streamline drug trials.[5]

It is likely that Callon and his colleagues may have drawn on knowledge of this period in the HIV/AIDS epidemic when they devised their model. Other historical accounts of HIV activism for drugs accord with Patton's sometimes citing of HIV/AIDS activism as having been a forerunner to a broader contemporary patient activism.[6] In sum, many would agree that the coming together of a mix of actors—gay activists, scientists, public policy analysts, medical practitioners—resulted in radical change in the rules of drug testing and, consequently, more rapid entry to the market of not just ARVs but other urgently required life-saving drugs.[7] Today, as the direct activism that initially infused HIV pharmaceutical innovation has been replaced by treatment information organizations, changing the rules of the game is a decidedly more "tame" process. The new mode of dealing with HIV is not directed toward seeking a sea change in the now-expanding field of HIV science, although there is activity toward gaining more investment in the development of vaccines and microbicides.[8] Instead, for the most part, effort is directed toward facilitating the best use of existing biotechnologies.

In practice, this means considerable effort is expended on dealing with the problems posed by ARVs, for example, attending to questions about which combination of drugs to choose, how to manage dosing adherence in an attempt to prevent drug resistance, and how to deal with iatrogenic disease or what are more often referred to as "side effects" of ARV. Textual material on these issues plays a critical part in achieving better understanding of the HIV biomedical field. It may consist of information on drugs disseminated by the pharmaceutical manufacturer. It may also include documented findings of a clinical study, medical notes from the clinic, conference papers, journal articles, or treatment information on the Web and in hardcopy magazines. The production of treatment information and also, as will be made apparent, the social science studies on difficulties posed by ARVs are aimed at bridging the gap between specialists and laypersons. But this is not all they do. In the process of reporting on drugs, they have a role in generating new knowledge and relations between members of the field. While the two areas of productivity—treatment information dissemination and research from the social sciences and humanities—are not usually regarded as having a direct relation to drug substance, they will be shown here to have direct input into pharmaceutical design.

The current capacity of treatment information disseminators and researchers in the social sciences to affect drug substance is consistent with yet also challenging of Callon and his colleagues' "hybrid forum." While the model put forward by Callon and his colleagues contests a monopoly view of the market by claiming that diverse interests and expertise forge the market dynamic and that consumers play an integral part in this, the model offers little insight into how historically differential workings of the dynamic are negotiated. That is to say, it does not recognize how the contributions of different actors may differ in force as well as content and that the interplay of interests may reflect this differential. Therefore, although I am keen to cast the HIV drug market according to the terms of the model of evolving hybrid activity, I also want to indicate the potential for different actors to influence an asymmetrical situation. In contrast to a conventional model that might assume monopoly control by pharmaceutical manufacturers or by pharmaceutical manufacturers and members of the discipline of science (here mainly chemistry) that is privileged as a source of authoritative knowledge, I focus on the potential influence of those less acknowledged or unacknowledged for their contributions to the forum. This will become clear as I pursue the very straightforward-seeming question: How might "consumer" input or representation be identified and used as a form of leverage in the struggle for better drugs?

The achievement of a satisfactory pharmaceutical response to HIV—frequently attributed to consumer activism, as I have already noted—is limited by iatrogenic disease effects as well as drug resistance. Indeed, the unsatisfactory nature of ARVs—and this is what I think may be the basis on which consumer leverage may be achieved—is a long way from what big pharma tells consumers they are entitled to expect. And since language plays an important role in the use of drugs, it also stands as a source for radical challenge. At its most insidious, language or text constitutes a domain of intelligibility that institutes a set of material givens or "material positivities" as if "outside discourse and power."[9] The logical corollary that follows from this argument is that material givens would be different in substance if language were directed differently. It is on these grounds that the role of language or the discursive is of special interest in the hybrid forum of ARVs. By highlighting the exchange of language I want to uncover the differential leverage some actors may have as they form part of an interdependent network. Further, taking a lead from Butler's argument on the role of language as it materializes and is therefore coextensive with our understanding of materiality,[10] I propose that different modes of textual expression be examined for their role in the substance of drugs. If I am correct in claiming that different modes of textual expression affect the substance of material interventions, then textual expression, in itself, becomes an important feature in a network reliant on textual exchange. To put this another way, if materiality is invariably an effect, at least in part, of the technologies—knowledges and hardware—it is possible to assume that textual expression in this process will play a significant role in the shaping of "the real" or "material."

## CASE STUDY: TRIZIVIR OR "THREE OLD IN ONE NEW"

Trizivir as a triple drug combination therapy was launched on the UK market in January 2001. However, it is important to note that the three drugs of AZT, Abacavir, and 3TC had been around for a number of years. New, then, was their incorporation into one pill, resulting in a reduction in the number of pills taken by the patient. The reduction of three pills into one was a significant advance for promotional purposes and also for some individuals grappling with the dosing difficulties of ARVs. Below, I trace out how this success was achieved through the contributions of non-corporate actors, including treatment information organizations. I also highlight how the campaign exceeded the confines of a juridical conception of language, that is, a conception of language as a transparent means of representation, which can be legislated upon as "true" or "misrepresentative." A reliance on this sort of juridical conception of language is evident in countries that impose regulatory mechanisms on drug development and marketing, for instance, the UK, the rest of the EU, and Australia.[11] It is presumed to protect the consumer against what some term "disease mongering," where misleading promotional tactics may cause members to believe they have a health condition that requires prescription drugs.[12] In my discussion of the UK Trizivir campaign I want to show that there is scope for considerably more play or reflexivity in how the language or, more specifically, the text of the actors involved comes to be embedded in drug substance. And that this exposes a too limited frame of reference in the assessment of "true" or "misleading" drug promotion.

### GSK's Trizivir

The expectations conveyed in the first person singular, in the advertisement in figure 3.1, appear to belong to a male, possibly in his mid-twenties or so. His shiny silver hip-hop puffer jacket, tortoiseshell-framed tinted serious-reading-style glasses, and hands-free mobile piece intend to convey a market-savvy individual. Cleverly stamped over his jacket is the GlaxoSmithKline (GSK) logo for Trizivir with what will become apparent as the repeated claim "Lives up to expectations." Across the image is the additional text "I expect my bank to rip me off. My mail to be on-line. And my HIV treatment to be ongoing. Not always on my mind." It is easy to read this fig-

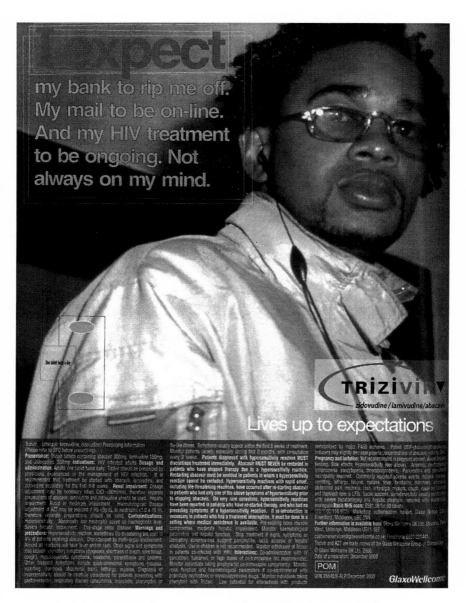

3.1     Color advertisement for Trizivir, manufactured by GlaxoSmithKline.

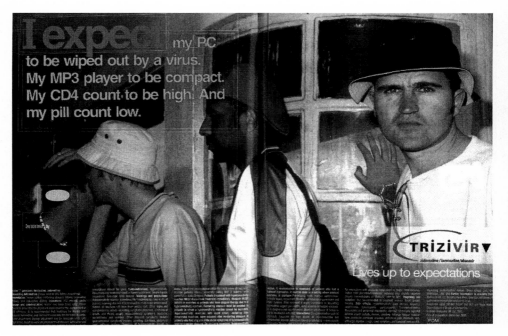

I expect my PC to be wiped out by a virus. My MP3 player to be compact. My CD4 count to be high. And my pill count low.

TRIZIVIR ▼

Lives up to expectations

3.2    Color advertisement for Trizivir, manufactured by GlaxoSmithKline.

ure of male embodiment, which is positioned a little higher than the camera and turned ever so slightly away, as a sign of confidence, self-certainty, and mobility.

In figure 3.2, another advertisement from the campaign shows a group of males similar in age to the man in figure 3.1. Particularly notable, in the original color version of figure 3.2, are the intense blue eyes of the individual facing the camera as they seem to squint back uncertainly: Too early in the day? Illicit behavior? It is hard to tell. The group beside him seems to be positioned in a loose queuing arrangement against a set of reflective windows or mirrors that might be found in the space of a late night or early morning clubbing scene. Interestingly, the last in the line faces away from the camera; his hand is wrapped around his head as if experiencing some anguish. The guy beside him whispers in his ear, leaving the viewer to guess at the content of the communication. The bold print over the image states: "I expect my PC to be wiped out by a virus. My MP3 player to be compact. My CD4 count to be high. And my pill count low."[13] And, again, the Trizivir logo with "Lives up to expectations." Both advertisements emphasize an ease of lifestyle available to those using Trizivir. Indeed, figure 3.2 suggests that Trizivir is so easy to use that it can be taken when out late at night or, perhaps to be more specific, can be incorporated in what the medical profession sometimes refers to as a "chaotic lifestyle," which may involve the use of recreational drugs.

For those who are familiar with HIV treatments, the mention of a high CD4 cell count in figure 3.2 will be recognized as the primary goal of ARVs. Familiar also will be the unstated but implicit need for strict dosing adherence in order to maintain drug levels for suppressing viral destruction of CD4 cells. It is these factors that made the low pill count—three drugs in one—Trizivir's key selling point. Since dietary restrictions have never been required for any of the three drugs that comprise Trizivir, the combination of the specific three-in-one pill continues to make it much more appealing than many other combinations. Yet while the advertisements tell the viewer of something significantly new to the market, those familiar with the medical history of ARVs will recognize shortcomings in the promotion that arise from the substance of Trizivir. For the drugs themselves—although easier to take in one pill and hence likely to help in reducing drug resistance through easier consistent dosing—are the "same old" and carry the same iatrogenic disease risks as they did prior to repackaging in Trizivir.

Bearing in mind what I have so far noted of the "good" and "bad" of Trizivir, and before I discuss how other media depicted Trizivir in the UK at its launch, I want to reiterate that these advertisements appeared in the UK context where direct to consumer (DTC) advertising of prescription drugs is prohibited. Therefore, while the above advertisements may look as if they were aimed at enlisting consumer self-identification, they were designed for a medical audience. I first came across them in an issue of the *Journal of Sexually Transmitted Infections*. They were brought to my attention by a specialist HIV clinician who remarked that his patients had asked him to prescribe Trizivir, in place of their existing regimen, after seeing it mentioned on television news.[14] This sort of request for a specific ARV combination would not be considered unusual were it not for the source that inspired it. People living with HIV include well-informed patients and many take an active role in determining their treatment. As mentioned above, their knowledge of available drugs comes from nonprofit treatment information dissemination organizations.[16] Interested by mention of an HIV ARV drug becoming known through mass-media news outlets, I began this study to see what it was that had captured such widespread attention and what this might suggest about the work of information in the biomedical management of HIV. For the clinician I spoke to and others I later came across, the advertisements did resemble a particular patient group, although these same practitioners expressed reservations about Trizivir, given the specific drugs comprising it and the availability of other more efficacious combinations.

In addition to the advertisements shown in figures 3.1 and 3.2, Trizivir was promoted with a publicity package (fig. 3.3) that has the image shown in figure 3.2 on its cover. The package—remarkably low-cost for a drug campaign—contained a series of information sheets (see fig. 3.1) with legislatively required information of known drug side effects plus GSK's own press sheet. Although it may not be surprising to learn that text from the package, including GSK's promotion text, reappeared in non-GSK media, it will serve as compound evidence of a textual hybridity that comes about through a commonplace yet relatively unexamined series of exchanges informing the HIV treatment field.

### News as Advertising—Another Actor for the Field

In promotional terms, Trizivir was able to acquire extensive media coverage that transgressed—remarkably, without contravening any law—the nationwide UK, and indeed EU, prohibition on direct-to-consumer (DTC) marketing of prescription drugs. The following headlines from major UK media outlets, specifically in London, appeared at the time of Trizivir's EU approval and its launch, two weeks later. They give weight to a certain type of newness and significant advance in the medical management of HIV promised by Trizivir. In fact, for those unaware of the risks of ARVs, it could seem that the destructive nature of the epidemic is past and, along with this, that large-scale public funding for research and prevention within wealthy nations with treatment access is no longer necessary:

"New HIV drug gets go ahead" (*The Times*, 4 January 2001)

"GSK Aids drug approved" (*The Times*, 5 January 2001)

"Health experts have welcomed the launch of the latest three in one HIV treatment" (Channel 5 News, 16 January 2001)

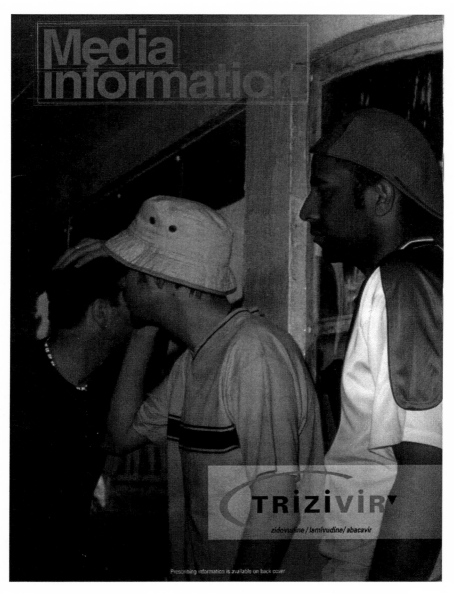

3.3    Color advertisement for Trizivir, manufactured by GlaxoSmithKline, on cover of publicity package.

"New anti-HIV pill is launched" (*The Independent*, 17 January 2001)
"User-friendly AIDS pill launched" (*The Metro*, 17 January 2001)

Despite the concern about direct drug promotion to the general public, it is not unusual for a drug to receive this sort of publicity and even to be proclaimed "a miracle drug."[16] Interestingly, it is also not usual for a news readership to be made aware that the text that leads to claims such as "consumer friendly" is provided through drug company copy. As would be expected then, the stories behind the above headlines varied only slightly. Indeed, there is a type of "clone" effect resulting from the way that the GSK publicity material was printed, possibly as intended and welcomed by GSK, without acknowledgment of its source. For example, *The Times* printed, without quotes, GSK's not unfounded claim that adherence was "one of the key challenges in tackling HIV infection." And both *The Metro* and *The Independent* printed a further GSK claim, again without quotes, that Trizivir is "designed to make it easier for people with HIV to treat themselves." At first glance, it might seem that this information is scientifically grounded and, therefore, that it comes from a GSK document need not be a concern. In light of these considerations, it is necessary to query, then, in what way this is different and necessarily disadvantageous to the coverage on Trizivir found, say, in refereed medical journals. Or, from a medical health perspective, if the statements are "scientifically correct," is there reason for concern? One response here might be that since this type of mainstream coverage is "news," not "advertising," it is likely to be presumed by a general audience to be more accurate or sufficiently so as not to involve the sort of critical reflection or at least "healthy" cynicism that advertising may induce. Hence, from this perspective, it could be said that mainstream news reporting provides a legitimizing effect for the HIV pharmaceutical industry.

Although news coverage, unlike advertising, can involve investigation of the product, in this instance there appears to be little difference in what was said by the pharmaceutical manufacturer and by authorized public media. This blurring of authorship highlights not only an exchange in which interests converge but, also, how the specific nature or work of some interests may be lost or muted in the process. Queries about the capacity of pharmaceutical products to meet consumer needs do not feature. This is largely to do with the function of scientific discourse, which enables big pharma interests to acquire dominance in the forum. As the privileged or master discourse in determining the legitimacy of drug text as well as drug substance—these are distinguished according to sign and matter—the capacity of scientific discourse to determine what can and cannot be said, as well as what is involved in the achievement of a pharmaceutical product, passes largely unchallenged. A drug may be questioned for whether its side effects have been accurately reported or whether it has been sufficiently tested according to government standards. But the enactment of a rational distinct disciplinary domain is rarely subject to question, the notable exception being the discipline of science and technology studies and to a considerably lesser extent the sociology of medicine.[17] Consequently, for the most part, the objects of science are presumed distinct from the vagaries of media coverage and other forms of input, to exist on the side of nature and not culture or flesh and not information.

## Medical and Consumer/Patient–led Treatment Media

The most expected sources for general information on a new drug or on a repackaged drug, whether for HIV or other conditions, are the broad-ranging journals for general medical practitioners. For this reason I want to add to my brief examination of media coverage of Trizivir, the coverage by the highly prestigious and widely read *British Medical Journal* (*BMJ*) and the similarly prestigious *Journal of the American Medical Association* (*JAMA*). Both frequently report on new drugs reaching the market. Indeed, entirely consistent with GSK publicity material, a *BMJ* editorial piece stated that Trizivir "is suitable for patients starting therapy or for whom adherence is a problem."[18] Although correct, the statement glosses over other issues posed by the combination including the likelihood that, for patients already on treatment, it may not be suitable due to its relatively high resistance profile and the potential for toxic side effects. Alluding to the more complex issues involved in assessing drug efficacy, *JAMA* provided a more detailed coverage of the treatment's pharmaceutical properties, its suitability, history of trials, and possible side effects, including hypersensitivity and lactic acidosis, which can be fatal, as well as severe liver problems, anemia, neutropenia, nausea, fatigue, and myopathy. Importantly, *JAMA* did not reiterate the GSK promotional emphasis on patient adherence for viral suppression but, instead, gave attention to the

fact that the drug had not been tested for maintaining long-term viral suppression in the presence of adherence.[19] It reinterpreted the GSK text suitable for the "therapy naive" and raised the more critical concern about how
well this combination might work over the long term, during which there is
increased chance of resistance developing from some drugs rather than others. That is to say, both *JAMA* and GSK—and so it might also be said of the
*BMJ*, if reflective of the anecdotal concerns expressed by practitioners that I
mentioned above—were aware that the market for Trizivir was likely to be
limited, simply because the individual drugs are proven as less efficacious
than others in overcoming viral resistance. Moreover, two years after the
Trizivir launch, this was confirmed. A trial in the United States was halted
after Trizivir was found less effective in treating "naive patients" than two
other combinations.[20]

### Entangled Interests

The dissemination of HIV treatment information in community-based
media conveyed the arrival of Trizivir and reflect a rather more diminished
set of expectations than those enunciated by GSK, as I show in the next section. Importantly the former's expectations appear considerably more low
key and less demanding of big pharma. To illustrate what I mean by this,
I have selected the Trizivir coverage in three HIV consumer-led treatment
information media sources: the online *HIV Treatment Bulletin*, *+ve Magazine*
online and in print, and *Positive Nation* magazine. Each gave mention to the
issue of adherence, which appears to be the marketing theme for Trizivir
and, as it seems, is reflected in Trizivir's pharmaceutical design.

The *HIV Treatment Bulletin* stated that "expected efficacy and risk related
to the 3 compounds" should be paramount, not ease of adherence.[21] Here
efficacy refers to the ability of the drug to suppress the virus, an issue already
noted above in discussion of the *JAMA* article and GSK's own publicity material. The *Bulletin* also referred to the ability of people to tolerate the combination in terms of side effects.[22] But, in spite of or because of the effort evident
here to assert a more independent and medically driven view, the reporting
also reflected and reinstated the way in which HIV treatments are phar-
macologically split. Ease of dosing for the subject is distinguished from the
body's need for the treatment. This is although, according to the science of

drug efficacy, the viability of subject and body is imbricated. While it is not within the remit of any treatment information organization to make "medical speak" accessible to a lay audience and, at the same time, deconstruct the presuppositions that inform this manner of speaking, the construction of a split subject/body warrants attention: How is it that the necessary act of dosing is assigned to self-directed agency and not also to physiological tolerability? For example, is it not possible that gagging—a reflexive physiological action—is beyond or other than such agency?

In contrast to the medically oriented critique in *HIV Treatment Bulletin*, *+ve Magazine* located itself at some political distance from the drug combination and its manufacturer through the use of cynicism. It stated: "Combining three drugs in a single tablet is being touted as an aid to adherence, because it reduces patients' pill burden."[23] But since no explanation was given for the use of the term "touted," the cynical register arguably did little to open debate. A more conceptually critical approach might have attended to the effects of a media heavily weighted toward delivery of the "facts." Even a cursory overview of HIV media at the time, as now, reveals the dilemma of the "informed patient" and raises the question of what sort of choices are required of this subject. While the GSK campaign suggests that choice and expectations of lifestyle are quite possible, constraints on therapies, such as hypersensitivity or drug resistance possible with Trizivir, suggest otherwise.

In addition to the coverage of Trizivir by *HIV Treatment Bulletin* and *+ve Magazine*, *Positive Nation* also mentioned Trizivir in terms of adherence. A half-page reduced black-and-white version of the two-page GSK promotion appeared in a regular section under the heading "Treatment News" (fig. 3.4). No text from the advertisement was included but, under it, was the following statement:

> They're the cover guys for the 16 January launch of Trizivir, GlaxoSmith-Kline's new three-drug combination pill. GSK says that combining AZT, 3TC and Abacavir in one pill enables three-quarters of patients to take their drugs correctly, compared with less than half taking a more complex regime. "Trizivir is a good choice for treatment of naive patients," said Dr. Margaret Johnson of London's Royal Free Hospital.[24]

Although the incorporation of the "news" item took place with an editorial identification of the source of the image, the dual role of Dr. Mar-

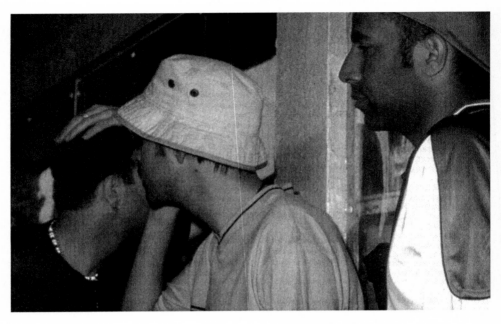

3.4 Edited version of figure 3.2, color advertisement for Trizivir, manufactured by GlaxoSmithKline, reproduced in black and white by *Positive Nation* magazine.

garet Johnson as a specialist HIV clinician and also in the service of GSK as part of the promotion is not mentioned.[25] While this omission may not have much bearing on a treatment-savvy audience—which, as I have noted, might be assumed of an HIV-positive readership[26]—the coverage could be claimed as lending itself to performing "promotional" if not "advertising" work for GSK. But, more useful, is to view the coverage as an example of a hybridity involving a merging of treatment information organizations and big pharma. While the two might be assumed to represent different, even competing, interests, it is apparent from the textual work of treatment information organizations that such organizations do not make this distinction.

Like medical practitioners, treatment information organizations must work with drug manufacturers. Both rely on drug manufacturers to inform them of pharmaceutical products and quite possibly to provide guidance for patients. And, in many instances, both medical practitioners and treatment information organizations receive drug company sponsorship.[27] This poses a series of challenges as funding is a necessary element for both areas. Nevertheless, it is important to point out that treatment information organizations would certainly not see themselves as swayed in their approach by this relationship. And sponsorship in return for drug advertising within treatment information material is usually rejected.[28] It is likely that *Positive Nation* reprinted the GSK advertisement and statement by Johnson on the presumption that all necessary procedures to guard against commercial interest, in contradistinction to patient-consumer interests, had already been addressed. On this basis I return to the "hybrid forum" of Callon and his colleagues and consider further the nature of an asymmetrical dynamic at work.

## Hybrid Dynamics in "Big Pharma" Reflexivity

As I indicated at the outset of this case study, despite the more than usual media coverage that took place before and at the time of Trizivir's release—equivalent to a breakthrough or advance in disease management—Trizivir as a combination therapy was already "old" prior to its promotion by *The Times* and *The Independent* newspapers as if "new." The three drugs that comprise it—Abacavir, Lamivudine, and Zidovudine—had been available for some time. In fact Zidovudine, best known as AZT, was the first anti-HIV drug of its type. And, although Trizivir is promoted as offering a treatment without dietary restrictions, as noted earlier, this was possible only because none of the three separate drugs require dietary restrictions. Small effort on the part of any mainstream media journalist might therefore have situated Trizivir in a different light from the unanimously enthusiastic response evident in the above headlines. Ironically though, as a result of the hype, it was also possible to claim that Trizivir did herald something new: a textual shift at the very least and one that was co-implicated in the repackaging of the treatment as three drugs in one pill.

The significance of this shift is illustrated in the coverage by the BBC Online News, which sought to offer a personal interest angle.[29] Consistent with the mainstream, medical, and consumer-led media line on adherence, a previously recalcitrant Craig Adams was quoted as claiming: "It means I will comply and adhere a lot more easily than I currently do."

In striking contrast to this self-surveillance, Dr. David Gordon, a medical advisor at GlaxoSmithKline stated:

HIV therapy is a fairly complex thing. We were asking patients to take a combination of usually at least three different drugs, and that often involves taking a large number of tablets with dietary restrictions. To get a true effect from these drugs you have to take almost all of them in the right way at the right time, and I think we were being a bit unrealistic in the past expecting patients to be able to comply and take these drugs entirely in the way that they were prescribed by doctors.[30]

Perhaps in response to published critiques of how patients continue to be positioned as failing drugs rather than drugs failing patients or, at least, the many studies that have identified adherence difficulties,[31] Gordon's statement could be read as a participant in, but also effect of, the hybrid dynamic, reflecting the merging of others' knowledge and expertise. Indeed this can be deduced from GSK's publicity package, the text of which appears to have provided the basis for much of the media coverage. Included in its text is a direct reference to a publicly funded social research report titled *Taking Heart* that focused on adherence difficulties from the perspective of an affected gay community.[32] It is hard to say whether those responsible for the report and whose research has shed valuable light on living with HIV pre- and now with ARVs, anticipated it would come to inform not just GSK's media but also its chemistry. For the purposes of this discussion, *Taking Heart*'s participation in this forum highlights the different ways knowledge can be put to work. Or, to put it another way, the use of *Taking Heart* by GSK is evidence of an exchange that may alter but, nevertheless, still partake in a terrain of uneven effects and differently valued interests. Its presence in the Trizivir text helps to show how Gordon's statement is a product of a hybrid space of HIV ARVs.

But this is not all that can be said of the statement, influenced as it is by *Taking Heart*, and likely by other social scientific studies on adherence difficulties. Discursively, if not also materially, the statement constitutes Trizivir as a liberating device, freeing the consumer-patient from the disruptive and difficult rigors of other dosing regimes. In doing so, it flips the expectation from that imposed on the subject of almost inevitable failure, to an expectation of drugs tailored to the subject's needs in work and leisure. The statement concurs with the GSK advertisements and can be argued to reveal a clever co-opting of forum interests to present GSK as acting in the interests of consumers. From a medical and consumer perspective, the development of Trizivir suggests that GSK has responded to the need for better design in terms of dosing requirements. From the perspective of the social theorist or cultural analyst, the GSK style of Trizivir marketing provides evidence of a highly contemporary textual play with significant bioethical implications.

Some of these bioethical implications are hinted at in the work of Kane Race, referred to in chapter 2. Noting that the emphasis on an HIV treatment "consumer" points to a new set of discursive effects being brought to bear on HIV identity, Race asks: "What happens when the HIV-positive are constituted as a niche market? What resistances and ruptures might this allow, in relation to the prior meanings and values attached to an HIV-positive identity?"[33] These questions anticipate some of what is evident in the innovative marketing style of GSK. Most certainly, they recognize the potential but also the incessant struggle that ARVs institute for those whose corporeality depends on them. The "freeing"-up from drug demands, on which the GSK promotional play depends, is not necessarily a trouble-free expectation. As Lisa Adkins points out in her work on labor market transformation, the very processes that involve detaching the individual from prior constraints effectively take place through the re-inscribing of such individuals—at the center of such processes—in new sets of rules, norms, and expectations.[34] The replacement of an onerous dosing regime with a simpler one is important but, in the case of Trizivir, it also involves taking on risks that may or may not apply to other drugs. In the GSK marketing of Trizivir, the person with HIV is portrayed as a consumer—confident, demanding, and, by implication, informed. As such he or she becomes the site to which responsibility for the management of the virus is shifted. This is despite the impossibility of the task, for it is fraught with the toxic effects of the drugs. Moreover, as Race points out, the overriding emphasis on not just adherence but, rather, its rationale, which is reduced viral load, privileges a surrogate measure of health over the experience of what might be termed "well-being" by the patient.[35] Is, then, managed viral load too singular a conception even when accompanied by a measure of CD4 cell count? Do diagnostics have more significance than "well-being" or "quality of life" when the potential toxic effects of the drugs remain, as termed, "side effects"?

## EXPECTATIONS—DO THEY NEED REVISING?

As I put together the material discussed above, I became increasingly aware of how big pharma construes itself as a valorized identity and, as in the Trizivir advertisements, expresses the latest populist concerns about health. Indeed, its branding engages with concerns about quality of life and, subtly, with possible public anxieties about corporate involvement in the health sector. For the big pharma Merck & Co., the current slogan is "Merck: Where patients come first."[36] For Bristol-Myers Squibb, the slogan is "At Bristol-Myers Squibb, our mission is to extend and enhance human life by providing the highest-quality pharmaceuticals and health care products."[37] For GlaxoSmithKline in the United States, the slogan is "GSK is a leader in serving communities in the US and around the world by discovering, developing and delivering innovative prescription medicines, vaccines, and other products that enable people to do more, feel better, live longer."[38] Without doubt the market that requires ARVs or other biomedical interventions comprises interests that big pharma must at least claim to serve in their competitive sphere. But these interests are themselves the consequence of a processual dynamic, that is, a network of exchanges over time. Hence these might continue to be affected—and more intentionally so—by those for whom they claim to speak. For instance, more demand by those engaged in deciphering the implications of ARVs or other biomedical interventions might call big pharma to account for its own chosen text, with the effect of mobilizing product design in ways more responsive to consumer needs. "Enhancing human life," "putting patients first," and "living longer" sound good but, as I have shown in the case of Trizivir, there is a worrying slippage in how these claims of big pharma interventions materialize.

While I do not want to deny the enormity of ethical responsibility attached to the role of the pharmaceutical industry, viewing it in terms of monopoly control may result in a form of assent to the most reductive agenda of big pharma: economic self-interest. By ceding all power to this industry, it is possible to lose sight of *how* corporate giants pursue market gain. In tactical terms, vital routes for how this pursuit might be re-directed or converted to allow for a more dynamic interplay of interests are closed off. Here I am suggesting that it is possible to see the HIV drug market as a dynamic entity consisting of many players or actors, a hybrid forum, while also seeing big pharma as centrally located in the orchestration of this. By conceiving of drugs as the achievement of numerous heterogeneous actors—inclusive of the body labor involved in synergizing the drugs and dealing with the virus—drugs become variable entities, embodying the work of many. Moreover, using the notion of "traffic," it becomes possible to see that the information passed on by different actors in the network or the "hybrid forum," in which interests transform each other, comes to be embedded in the substance or molecular design of a drug. Information as the text of drugs is, then, a force or line of flight, as Deleuze and Guattari might say, in the making of the molecular. That is, it is a rupture creating new potential in a network of actors and their relations with each other.[39]

The textual use of "expectations" in GSK advertising begs the question of why the elimination of toxic effects is not included among these expectations. What sort of priorities are at work in drug design that ease of adherence comes to be weighed against long-term suppression and toxic side effects? And how, it may also be important to ask, does the subject/body split function, such that a choice between these differentiated aspects of treatment emerges as a key dilemma? Whether treatments make HIV an insignificant factor in everyday life may well depend on ease of dosing but also on what they do to the body and the virus. Incorporating treatments into daily life is unlikely to be a consideration distinct from others—namely, drug efficacy and side effects—if the exercise of choice is constituted within the limits of "life threatening." To return specifically to the difficulties of treating and ultimately eradicating the damage of the virus and drugs, the following question might be asked: If, within the remit of any anti-HIV pharmaceutical manufacturer, the consumer's needs are the priority and treatments are intended as a response to these needs, as GSK has claimed, is it time to do more than just reduce the number of pills to be swallowed?

Through a clever promotional campaign, GSK could be said to have contested some of the constraints placed on the highly regulated subject of the clinic, namely difficult dosing regimes. It could also be said that the move by GSK to devise a combination drug therapy that fits drug taking into patients' lifestyles—an argument put forward by clinicians and social researchers—is indicative of a company intent on an image of being responsive to clinicians and consumer-led organizations.[40] Yet, irrespective of the validity of this intent, by repackaging AZT, Abacavir, and 3TC into Trizivir, as just one pill, GSK has shown that ARVs may be more malleable than otherwise thought and, as a consequence, that there is more to be said of and demanded in drug design. Indeed, GSK has unwittingly created a specific area for redress by bringing into relief the unhappy split between what the individual subject may want from life and the requirements of his or her body.

## CONCLUSION

In the case study that I have presented, the process of exchange that is active in constituting both the knowledge and the substance of drugs is confined to one particular ARV, Trizivir. This antiretroviral treatment combination and the text informing and following from it has been especially useful to highlight the hybrid forum in which a dynamic interplay of knowledge and substance takes place. Although big pharma is assumed to be driven by an interest in gaining a greater share of the ARV market, this invariably involves the contributions of others, namely people living with HIV, their clinicians, scientific and social scientific researchers, social critics of HIV, and highly sophisticated treatment information dissemination organizations. But Trizivir has also been valuable for highlighting the unevenness of this exchange. It is claimed by its manufacturer to address consumer needs, but only as these needs are hived off—in the text and as substance—from the material constraints posed by HIV and/or ARVs. The achievement of an "everyday" lifestyle requires being free of not only the onerous demands of dosing schedules but the demands of infection and drug toxicity. From this point of view, there is a very clear need to find ways of instating more expansive expectations or reappropriating existing ones in the synergy of interests that is drug substance.

My approach has been tied to a historic shift or, indeed, transformation, in the field whereby treatment information organizations have come to replace the activists of a pre-ARVs period. Although I fully support the contribution made by those who enable patients and their doctors to be more informed of drug combinations and their implications, I also want to see more use made of their work. While identified—indeed, self-identified—with the point of ARV consumption, possibilities for a more directed input into the production process are easily overlooked. This point may be similarly applied to social researchers. Study of the impact of ARVs on clinical expectations and, most especially, on dosing adherence can also facilitate new approaches by big pharma as the latter aspires to access niche markets with the claim of addressing consumer needs. It is not difficult to make the claim that ARVs are unsatisfactory for meeting the needs of people with HIV and, not surprisingly, irrespective of what ARV advertising may imply or even when it seems that direct advertising is prohibited and therefore assumed absent. Text is one means for tackling this. As I have argued, advertising need not be ignored or considered as merely a textual production for regulation and largely by restriction. The Trizivir campaign—although relatively low cost with its card package of contemporary lifestyle images and juridically accurate reporting on adherence and side effects—has shown that media may morph. By moving away from a juridical conception of restriction and classical realist ideas of representation—with their presumption of a material given—it becomes possible to rethink the use of text. Reliance on the juridical and realist view of information as potentially misleading and to be prohibited or restricted misses the point, or at the least the big point. While big pharma has shown itself able to take advantage of traffic in information and flesh—such that information becomes flesh—the rest of us may be left behind. In this instance, what initially began as advertising within a nondirect consumer context was able to permeate the highly legitimized vehicles of news reports. But more importantly, it was already part of an acquiring of the market through the co-option of non-pharma labor in bringing to light the difficulties of dosing.

As a final note, I want to add that while my focus has been on the question of lifestyle in the context of an enabled consumerist culture and is very much directed in analytic style to contexts where ARVs are readily available, the argument put forward should be considered also for its relevance to those patients without access to ARVs. For along with the political and economic explanations for the forestalling of ARVs in countries such as those comprising sub-Saharan Africa, there are the critical issues of viral resistance and iatrogenic disease.[41] In other words, without diminishing in any way the urgency to mobilize access to ARVs in resource-poor contexts, the complex and damaging dimensions of ARVs are part of this mobilization. They underscore the urgent need to harness big pharma interests in response to articulated concerns of the non-big pharma participants. This is not only in relation to questions of drug provision and drug delivery but, also, in relation to the design of drugs whose iatrogenic risks require extensive infrastructure prior to, in many instances, appropriate provision and delivery.

# 4

# THE "INFORMED MATTER"
# OF HIV PREVENTION

I N THE INTRODUCTION TO THIS BOOK I REFERRED TO THE WAY THE ADVENT
of antiretroviral therapies forged a decoupling of HIV from AIDS. In the
previous chapters I have suggested that this decoupling is the matter of a
significantly altered epidemic. Here I focus on what this might be understood to mean for HIV prevention, concentrating on gay-identified men as
the long-term target of prevention in the history of the epidemic. In contexts
of full treatment access with concentrated epidemics among gay men, medical interventions have altered not only the virus, as discussed in chapter
2, but also the complex assemblage that is prevention. To put this another
way, while HIV continues to be the focus of those working and living with
the epidemic, it and what might be assumed to be the objects associated
with it—subjects, bodies, and knowledges—have altered. In social research
attuned to an increasingly medicalized epidemic, the alteration is likely to
be characterized as a series of shifts in risk understandings and practices. For
the most part I want to revise this characterization as it tends to presume
that the target of prevention is an individual within, yet *apart from*, a context of knowledges and biomedical interventions. Although this view can be
argued to have been effective prior to ARVs, I suggest that a more relational
account of risk will be more responsive to a biomedically altering field.

At the time ARVs were introduced, science gave promise that infection
rates resulting from unsafe sexual practice could be reduced as a consequence of reduced individual viral loads.[1] That is, on the basis that ARVs
would reduce the "pool" of virus available for transmission, it was conjec-
tured that rates of infection would decrease. Treatment was viewed as a
potential aid to prevention and, it is possible to add, a relation of sorts—
limited to a conception of the biological—was recognized to exist between

treatment and prevention. But despite the reduced "pool," infection rates remain the same or, more worryingly, in some places have increased.[2] By the early 2000s, confirmation that unprotected anal intercourse (UAI) had become more commonplace for some gay men in the presence of ARVs, and that this has led to an increase in new infections, provoked many to query the sustainability of current HIV prevention.[3]

In response to the unanticipated rise in infections, considerable debate has taken place about the relationship between the presence of ARVs and potentially risky sexual practice.[4] To gain more insight into this relationship and most especially on how risk and, inferred with this, responsibility for prevention are now conceived among gay sexual communities, various qualitative as well as quantitative studies have been and continue to be carried out.[5] Indeed my initial research into HIV involved a study conducted with Kane Race and Susan Kippax in 1999 and 2000 that provides the material discussed in the final sections of this chapter.[6] Our finding at the time took into account the explanation of "treatment optimism" affecting attitudes and practices, but located this as part of a changing context resulting in a more fractured or diverse community of gay men.[7] Working closely with community organizations and gay-affiliated advisors to government, we reached the conclusion that knowledge of ARVs and associated tests provides the conditions of possibility for some gay men to devise more inventive and varied risk-reduction sexual strategies—although not necessarily always successful—than those authorized by public health campaigns pre-ARVs.[8]

Later in the chapter I rework the idea that biomedical technologies provide a condition of possibility for what is often termed within the HIV prevention field gay men's "risk calculus."[9] Although I do not want to dispense with the idea that a phenomenon such as altered risk calculus emerges out of a set of conditions, I do want to develop the idea in a manner that overcomes an implicit distinction between the human target of prevention and everything else that might be considered to affect whether infection takes place. For the most part, and reflected to some extent in my own earlier research, assessments of biomedical intervention in reference to prevention tend to be underpinned by a conception of risk that is attached to the work of an individual human. As I mentioned in the introduction when illustrating PEP (post-exposure prophylaxis), biotechnologies are viewed as "tools" whose effects—intended or otherwise—follow from the ideas or information held by those who may or may not use them in relation to risk. While this facilitates research into human practices, it installs a given and therefore normative conception of human agency as distinct from the matter that it is affecting and affected by. Consequently, the potential within this co-constitutive relationship to advance more effective prevention is largely unexplored. Within the HIV field, the normative idea of human-centered agency finds direct expression in debates on whether to make post-exposure prophylaxis available to HIV-negative gay men at risk of infection. For it is feared that the publicizing of this biotechnology will enable them to reconsider their practice of safe sex (anal intercourse with condoms) and, on this basis, some members of the public health field argue *against* the provision of the biotechnology.[10]

The focus on human agency and the consequent proclivity towards restricting, if not withholding, a prevention technology is not surprising given the range of studies to investigate changes in sexual practice that imply—since the introduction of ARVs—that gay men have become "complacent" and display a poor or deficient attitude to risk.[11] But, as Race has argued, a very different explanation of change becomes necessary through only brief reflection on the history of the epidemic. Behavior change involving the take-up of condoms or other forms of risk minimization by gay men as a response to HIV risk has, from the outset, involved what Race describes as "reflexive mediation between embodied habits and medical opinion."[12] This mediation is shown to have long involved incorporation of medical knowledges into practice (indeed since the days when infections were first identified among gay men) and in ways that have sustained gay culture. Hence, in Race's schema and following on from our earlier research emphasizing the contributory role of biomedical innovation, gay men's agency is recast as creatively achieved rather than negatively measured against an imagined norm. In other words, the idea of a human subject wrongly enabled by "treatment optimism" is evidence of a field too tied to the presumption of gay men behaving badly and to the exclusion of a more dynamic account of prevention as an assemblage of "informed matter." To illustrate what I mean by this, and indicate the increasing importance of moving beyond the distinctions of human and biotechnology or even human subject and body prevalent in current prevention approaches, I show how the gay male individual of HIV prevention efforts is an historical and diverse entity who embodies—in varying ways—the dynamic context against which more conventional approaches would situate and fix him. Although enacted and self-enacting according to the neo-liberal notions of agency and responsibility, self-identified gay men need to be seen as much more than and different from this.

## AN ALTERNATIVE ANALYTIC: INFORMED MATTER

To allow for a more dynamic field of activity—in which onus for HIV is redistributed across the field to encompass the design of biomedical technologies and the revision of current interventions—I want to appropriate a concept of "informed matter," as coined by Andrew Barry in an argument on the nature of pharmaceutically invented molecules. Although work on molecules may seem altogether too tangential, the notion of "informed matter" provides a novel way for rethinking biomedicalized or newly technologized prevention. Hence I will extend this concept to help characterize HIV prevention as an assemblage of sorts that delivers up the prevention target of a sexually active gay man.

Paraphrasing an article by Bernadette Bensuade-Vincent and Isabelle Stengers on "informed materials," Barry states in reference to the inventiveness of chemical research and development: "Molecules should not be viewed as discrete objects, but as constituted in their relations to complex informational and material environments."[13] In contrast to conventional scientific thought—where there is some "thing" or, as Barry states "a set of given possibilities out of which effective drug molecules can subsequently be synthesized"—Barry enables us to see that atoms and molecules are always already enmeshed in an association or set of relations; that is, molecules are not there waiting to be discovered but emerge through a context of relational differences.[14] The argument is developed from the work of A. N. Whitehead, who viewed chemistry as a science of associations of atoms and molecules and argued, as Barry explains: "A molecule should be considered an historical rather than a physical entity. Molecules certainly endure, but it cannot be assumed that they remain the same." This is because, as Whitehead stated: "physical endurance is the process of continuously inheriting a certain identity of character transmitted throughout an historical route of events."[15] The process is the *making* of the entity or, to turn this around, the entity is the effect of a process of relations or associations: "how an actual entity becomes constitutes what [*sic*] that actual entity is."[16] Important, then, is that entities may be considered ontologically different when formed on different occasions. For Barry, a molecule will have a different identity and produce different effects in a laboratory than in the body. Moreover, in the specific environment of pharmaceutical research and design, information is built *into* the structure of the molecule.[17] This "information" may include data about potency, metabolism, and toxicity but, also, intellectual property law, patents, and other legal or economic information. In this way, the molecule embodies its environment or, as Barry puts this: "an environment of informational and material entities *enters into* the constitution of an entity such as a molecule."[18]

The idea that an entity embodies its environment and, as I shall suggest later, is involved in a co-constitutive relationship with its environment, will be used here to devise a supplementary methodological approach to the ARV information-rich context of prevention. Staying with the notion of the gay sexually active male as the target of intervention but unsettling the way in which making him responsible for transmission leaves out other aspects involved in "his" negotiations with HIV, I shall propose a different entity of prevention. Featuring in this will be sex. Sex can be understood as a remarkably enduring and changing feature of the epidemic: not only as a source of transmission but also as a source of the most conceptually and materially effective intervention. Its potential as such resides in its performance or enactment in and through a host of relations—not simply human relations but relations involving non-human actors: condoms, HIV antibody testing, and virus. These and more—including the meshing of place, "body language," attachment, and anonymity—contribute to its dynamic nature in relation to HIV.

## "IN YOUR FACE": DISENABLING TECHNOLOGIES OF IDENTITY (A WHILE BACK)

The focus of this section is on how sex has been a contested site in the course of the epidemic. Most inventively, in association with gay sexuality, sex was reworked early on in the epidemic well before the advent of ARVs to limit the traffic of HIV.[19] Indeed, the carefully choreographed way in which gay men have developed a culture of safe sex has been the mainstay of effective prevention in countries within Western Europe, in Australia, New Zealand, and North America.[20] The following brief outline of a pre-ARV context and the importance of sex then, as now, will offer some insight into the historically rich and, it could be added, heterogeneous context now diversely *embodied* in gay sexual cultures illustrated in the concluding section.

> A condemnation to celibacy or death
> God's punishment for our weaknesses
> God's test of our strengths
> The price paid for the 1960s
> The price paid for anal intercourse
> The result of moral decay and a major force destroying the Boy Scouts
> Nature's way of cleaning house

The above phrases are recorded in the now well-known essay by Treichler, "AIDS, Homophobia and Biomedical Discourse: An Epidemic of Signification." The variation and, at times, contradictions in the list I have extracted from a far longer one compiled by Treichler will give some sense of the ways in which mass media, in association with the United States government and sections of the Christian (including Catholic) churches, represented people infected with HIV. Explicit or implicit is the claim that people with HIV brought it on themselves through "wrongful" or "unnatural" acts. This mode of constituting HIV as a disease of victims who suffer as a consequence of their own or their society's moral failure—conflating sexuality and disease—was reflected in the Reagan administration's refusal to speak of HIV/AIDS when the virus was first identified. Some argue that the administration's early silence led to many millions of deaths. By 1985, when the Reagan administration finally recognized the need for a public health policy, over 12,000 Americans had been diagnosed with AIDS, over 6,000 had died, and the epidemic had already expanded within the United States and in sub-Saharan Africa.[21] In contrast, governments in countries such as the United Kingdom, Canada, and Australia responded more immediately to the crisis by supporting the development of prevention education, establishing medical services (mainly palliative care wards), and, in some instances, introducing legislation in an endeavor to protect those affected by HIV from discrimination. Nevertheless, the broad influence of the United States plus a preexisting homophobia, post-colonial Eurocentrism, and blatant racism across much of the international spectrum can be understood as integral to an epidemic where what was said and what was not facilitated the transmission of HIV.[22]

In response to the transmission spreading approach of the Reagan era and of other political conservative groups, a most extraordinary activism emerged within gay and lesbian communities across the globe. Frequently this involved especially strident assertions or subversions of forms of sex and sexuality that were provocative with intended political force. The material I have selected is from an exhibition staged at the National Gallery of Australia in 1994 titled Don't Leave Me This Way: Art in the Age of AIDS. The close relationship between the Australian government and gay communities made possible a display of individual and community art gathered from all over the world. In the words of its curator Ted Gott, the exhibition reflected "the onslaught of HIV/AIDS on the personal, social, moral and political fabric of Western societies." For Gott, Don't Leave Me This Way provided a space for artists to "speak to, empower and educate their audiences in the widest sense."[23] The audience in this context included those most directly affected, but also those requiring adjustment in their too ready acceptance of HIV/AIDS as a disease affecting "Others." The works I have selected from the exhibition may be noted for their willful use of explicit sexual themes, aimed at countering the demonizing of gay sexuality that construed those living with HIV and dying from AIDS as tragic passive victims or, in Butler's words, as if "the less 'human.'"[24] In some instances, material from the exhibition can be said to have marked the early stages of queer theory and its transcendence of normative identity politics that I draw on to query the performative work of clinical trials in chapter 5.

## Don't Leave Me This Way . . .

The three photographs, Mark I. Chester's "Robert Chesley —ks portraits with harddick & superman spandex" #1, #3, and #5 from a series of 6 images, "Diary of a Thought Criminal," San Francisco, 1989 (fig. 4.1)[25] and Jamie Dunbar's *Posithiv Sex Happens* (fig. 4.2), can be viewed as interventions in the struggle to contest popular media portrayals of people with HIV/AIDS. In

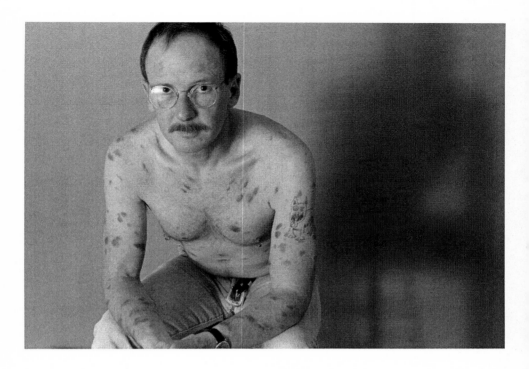

4.1   Mark I. Chester, United States, "Robert Chesley —ks portraits with harddick
      & superman spandex #1, #3, #5, from a series of 6 images, "Diary of a Thought
      Criminal," San Francisco, 1989, gelatin silver photographs. Courtesy of the artist.

contrast to the reducing of people with HIV/AIDS to no more than their disease, these works ask the viewer to reflect on their own practice of looking.

In reference to the full series of Chester's work on Chesley, Jan Zita Grover provided the description: "bare-chested, his torso covered with Kaposi's
sarcoma legions, in his Superman fetish costume—*a fully sexual person with
AIDS*" [my emphasis].[26] In a critique not dissimilar from Douglas Crimp's
commentary on media images and the project of ACT UP (AIDS Coalition
to Unleash Power) to convey a person not reduced to the abject of disease,[27]
Grover goes on to state:

> Chester's portrait series explored Chesley's body as a site marked not only by
> disease but by desire. These are issues that people living inside the contradic-
> tions of HIV/AIDS may be driven to explore and resolve in what is often a

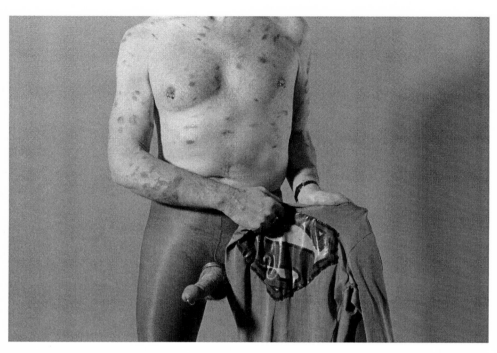
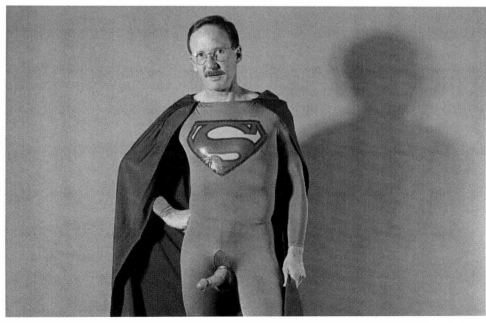

flow of images, as if no single photograph could contain the complexity of the journey or destination.[28]

In the subversive style of queer, it is possible to read the images as a refusal by gay men to slip quietly out of view, forever; and as performing precisely what would otherwise drive them from view by their "immoral, ungodly behaviour." Chesley's ease in looking intentionally at camera, while marked by disease through the visually evident Kaposi's sarcoma (KS), a form of cancer common to those with AIDS, and marked by his sex, demands a type of double take. This embodied desiring subject challenges the familiar everyday way we have come to expect to see or not to see sex: not only do the subject and artist refuse to relegate their sexual desire to the closet, they use rhetorical play through reference to the figure of "Superman," the figure who must always transcend his "closeted" alter ego Clark Kent. Stripped down to his spandex Superman suit—a figure of vigor with disease—Chesley could be read as standing also for the public good. By bringing together the otherwise jarring elements—of sex, disease, and savior—he functions as a transgressive performative of pleasure despite disease. That is, he refuses to be reduced to a pathology of disease, objectified and, in being so, refused viability. Both photographs exceed the boundaries of what might otherwise constrain desire, not only in terms of "who" we desire but "how" we desire. The "out" of the "harddick" is crucial here. Don't Leave Me This Way becomes a demand, a maximizing of what might also be read as phallic force gone awry, no longer in the service of hetero-ness.

Similar to the Chester work, in Jamie Dunbar's *Posithiv Sex Happens* (fig. 4.2) this studio image refuses the more usual relegation of infection as an object for cordoning and also the way in which medicalized spaces, notably those of the hospital—here marked by the intravenous drip—are complicit in this. Medical intervention is utilized here against its more usual sectioning-off of sex from the constituted space of treatment and, significantly, against the otherwise death-inducing work of exclusion from treatment that was taking place at the time. The two bodies in this image embrace in a manner that recasts medicine as having the capacity to be "life serving," rather than "life saving" or "life preserving." Viability is linked to sexual vitality, as if co-constitutive of each other and *Posithiv* comes to be enacted as both value and medical condition. Indeed, while bodies are here overtly linked to a

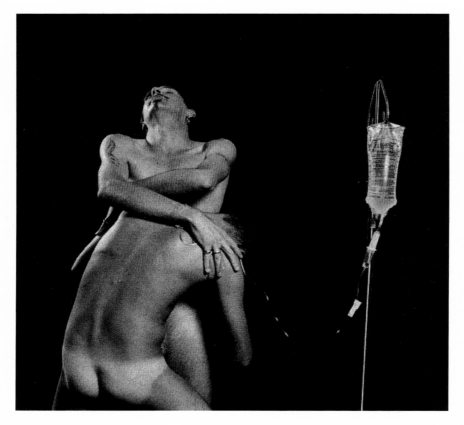

4.2   Jamie Dunbar, Australia, *Posithiv Sex Happens* 1993, gelatin silver photograph.
      Courtesy of the artist.

"life-sustaining medical technology" and overtly sexualized in their relation
to this technology, it is the sexualization of the medical technology that is
most provocative.

   In contrast to these formalized photographic pieces were materials more
explicitly intended to contribute to HIV prevention education. Of these I
have selected a poster by David McDiarmid, which was commissioned by
the AIDS Council of New South Wales, Australia, and used as part of its
education campaign for safe sex (fig. 4.3). At the center of the Australian
campaign was a commitment to work with gay sexual communities to institute the use of condoms in ways that supported gay sexual cultures stricken

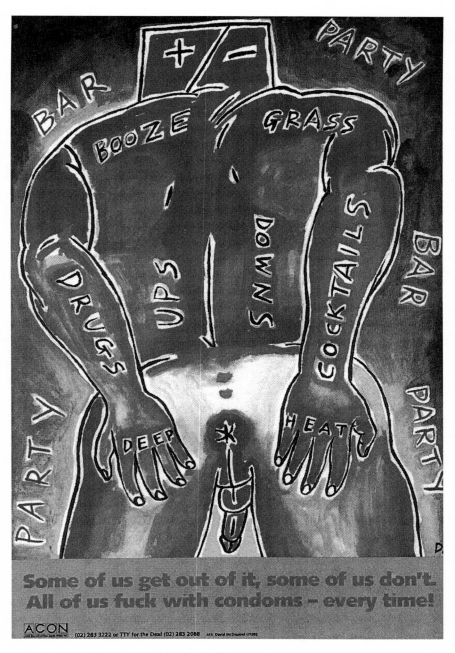

4.3 David McDiarmid, Sydney, Australia, produced for the AIDS Council of New South Wales, *Some of US Get Out of It, Some of US Don't. All of Us Fuck with Condoms—Every Time!* 1992, offset lithography. National Gallery of Australia, Canberra, gift of AIDS Council of New South Wales.

by the virus. A retrospective of McDiarmid's work included a statement by him explaining:

> I wanted to do something that would still be pro sex . . . when you are doing a safe sex poster there isn't room for ambiguity. Your message has to be crystal clear.[29]

Commentary with the retrospective noted:

> While the recent rise [in UAI and infection rates] poses questions about the need for new strategies of refreshment in education and prevention, Australia's success historically in dealing with HIV/AIDS is remarkable.

The last statement refers to Australia's outstanding record in reducing its rate of HIV transmission. It was elaborated by another on how government action was able to "save the lives of thousands of people (gay and straight) and avoid the social and political backlash against gay rights that seemed for a time to be imminent."[30] McDiarmid's posters did not just aim to be explicit and unambiguous, though. They played on a certain sharp, provocative, "in your face" wit of a culture railing and rallying against unspeakable loss and suffering.

Provocation was immensely important and McDiarmid's posters along with other aesthetic interventions such as Chester's and Dunbar's helped to create a sense of gay "community" through which, prior to ARVs, condoms became normalized in gay men's thinking and practice of anal intercourse. While it is important to note that this exceptional change to sexual practice occurred in a context of a publicly visible disease presence and, for many gay men, the loss of friends and lovers, the take-up of condoms remains extraordinary as a strategy. Anal intercourse was sustained without, for most, the transmission of HIV and, for the most part, without the otherwise likely occurrence of stigma and discrimination against people with HIV. People were encouraged to function as if members of a sexually homogeneous community, not divided in their social and or sexual relations by HIV positive and negative status. The associated elements that changed sexual practice have forged a historically enriched environment not just constitutive of but embodied in some gay men as the target of prevention.

## BIOMEDICALIZED SPEECH

I'm including here only a few of the interview extracts provided by self-identified gay men from the study I conducted with Race and Kippax in Australia between 1999 and 2001,[31] but they will be sufficient to illustrate some of the ways that the altered virus now works in not just the minds or the bodies of gay men but in a manner that requires holding at bay a distinction of minds and bodies. Further, while these are texts in the conventional sense of having been produced from spoken interviews and transcribed onto the page, they are read here as expressions of an historic route or process of endurance and change.[32] And cast as such, they provide access to a relational process in which information and flesh may be understood to have mixed to effect new properties embodying and affecting changed times.

Most of the extracts are from HIV-positive men who agreed to discuss their decision to practice sex without condoms. The phrase "sex without condoms" is used here in place of UAI, as it will be evident in the first quote below that sex is a more diverse practice than just anal intercourse. It should also be evident from the material that anal intercourse without condoms is not necessarily "unsafe" or at least not necessarily unsafe when risk considerations work as intended. Later in the discussion, an additional interview is included with a HIV-negative man who had received PEP (post-exposure prophylaxis involving a month's course of ARVs) and whose comments offer further insight into how biomedical knowledge is meshed with bodily phenomena.

> I'm really upfront about my status and if someone wants to have unprotected sex . . . It's not an issue um really, in a lot of ways. I tend to be a receptive partner if you're just talking about fucking . . . what I like in sex is pretty broad. So, fucking . . . most probably used to be fairly major and now it's not so major. . . . I'm not good at stats and figures, but there's a much higher chance of him [negative partner] becoming infected if I come inside him as opposed to the other way around . . . I also wonder about viral load levels, you know. I know viral load tests only measure the virus in blood and—it [HIV] could be higher in other parts of the body—but . . .

To a reader unfamiliar with the significance of the viral load test in the clinical management of HIV, it may not be apparent from the above that the interviewee, Tim, who is HIV-positive, had a constant viral load recorded measurement of "undetectable." Nevertheless, it is possible to deduce this from his suggestion that "it could be higher in other parts of the body," which implies the presence of a test and one that cannot be assumed to represent viral measure in semen. It is also important to note from his statement that his sexual practice is not what would be considered high risk by epidemiological estimates. Much of it may include practices that do not involve penis/anus intercourse. Further, when engaging in UAI, he is the receptive (non-penetrating) partner, which is epidemiologically low risk to a negative insertive partner.[33] It may also be helpful to know that he stated in the course of his account that ARVs had brought about an improvement in his state of health and emotional being that, as he put it, made it possible for him to consider having sex.

From a prevention point of view, the possibility of avoiding infecting a partner, an ARV-improved body and emotional state, plus adoption of the receptive position or what has been termed "strategic positioning" could be read as an inventive approach to "risk calculus."[34] This reading would not be at odds with the additional reading that Tim's stated practice is the product of "AIDS fatigue,"[35] a fatigue that comes from adhering to safe sex[36] messages likely to have been heard by him for over twenty years. Nor would such a reading be at odds with the possibility that Tim's revised conduct reflects "treatment optimism" about the effectiveness of ARVs in preventing AIDS.[37] Indeed, by combining Tim's related conduct (receptive position when engaging in anal intercourse) and state of health ("undetectable" viral load), it is possible to conceive of him as a gay subject formed through HIV/AIDS prevention messages and epidemiological risk estimates. In sum, the text provided here conveys a speaking subject who distinguishes between some practices and others. It is made possible through the enactment of the HIV antibody test and the viral load test. Hence, something that might be developed with Barry's account of informed matter is the relational nature of a context becoming embodied in the human body of surveillance. The body emerges through a process of enrichment in properties, including a reduction in virus and alteration in sexual practice. But it might also be said that there is a dynamic process at work. It involves a newly technologized and, importantly with this, an ontologically different human subject or, indeed, multiple ontological subjects constitutive of their environment.[38]

Tim's becoming ontologically different post-ARVs is not simply forged through the work of signs such as viral load counts—metaphysical absence—but, on the contrary, through a fleshed engagement with these flesh informed diagnostics as well as ARVs. In particular, the viral load test materializes a reading of "undetectable," which is more than knowledge in the sense that it has already involved a collaboration or intra-action of body matter, virus, and the matter that comprises the test. "Undetectable viral load," or even "HIV positive" or "HIV negative" status, are not mere "knowledge" in the sense of distinct from the flesh. They are, if we are to accept bioscience, a state of flesh. Tim's subjectivity—in particular, his speaking and acting—is the effect of an embodied engagement with biomedical technologies. He is, as Barry might argue, his enriched environment. Indeed, on the basis of what he says "an environment of informational and material entities" can be said to have *entered into* his being and into his deliberated enacted negotiation of viral presence with a partner in sex. No doubt he exhibits agency in his doing, but as a doer he embodies much of what has taken place in the course of the epidemic by HIV prevention educators, gay activists, and scientists. Moreover, his doing is part of the performing and transforming of a wider environment.

In the following extract, Ian, also HIV-positive and chronologically older than Tim but having seroconverted (become HIV antibody positive) after the advent of ARVs, also conveys something of an inventive "risk calculus." Finding himself HIV-positive was, he indicates, a profound challenge to his existence in the world and, as he also indicates, instituted a different way of being:

> I went through a huge depression for a while and didn't have sex probably for nine months and didn't think I ever would, you know, it [becoming HIV-positive] was the end of the world. I wasn't sick so . . . and I realised I wasn't probably going to be sick for a while and I might even live. Gradually I started going out again . . . it was a long time before I ventured back into the ordinary world and thought of having sex with somebody who is either negative or I didn't know . . . I got a bit militant about it for a while. I'd thought I'll only ever fuck somebody who is positive. I feel I have a duty not to put somebody at risk, you know. . . . But I feel quite differently, you know, about it all and certainly than I did before.

Ian went on to indicate that condoms are a significant factor in his decision to practice UAI:

> I find them [condoms] obstructive. I quite often lose a hard-on with them. I don't feel the same sensation . . .

To deal with this, Ian recounts a strategy of serosorting (where partner selection is based on sharing the same HIV antibody status), which is aimed at avoiding condoms and involves reading the signs of a potential partner:[39]

> I never elect to use them [condoms]. I don't force myself on anyone either. If I don't know them then I don't know their status. I usually will not try and initiate to fuck them or to be fucked by them without initiating some sort of conversation . . . not necessarily about status, but about whether or not someone wants a condom. I won't just let it [sex with risk] happen . . .

Not just letting it happen requires some familiarity with the sexual culture of which Ian understands himself to be a part. A certain familiarity or skill is evidently necessary to establish agreement for UAI with a partner while avoiding discussion of serostatus. That is, it is possible to read Ian's strategy as seeking a partner of the same serostatus but without putting this into speech. In part only it reflects the sort of prevention campaigns referred to earlier and captured in the poster by McDiarmid. Such prevention campaigns emphasized nondisclosure of serostatus to avoid possible discrimination against HIV positive men and, also, possible false claims of negative serostatus that could lead to transmission. But their central message was that condoms be used in every sexual encounter. Alternatively, Ian's strategy could be read as aiming to obtain consensual UAI, without necessarily relying on serosorting. Whichever reading is made, it is apparent that Ian's bodily practice is historically informed and in ways that challenge a stable distinction between social knowledge and bodily practice. The body is not only interpreted through his own informed HIV status. It is read in ways that accord with how his informed status is relational to a fleshed other. When asked on what occasions he would use a condom, Ian said:

You make assumptions about the way they [people in venues] present themselves, the way they behave in there, their body language. I make assumptions that they're negative if they look a bit green or uncertain or unsure of
themselves, or they don't look, you know, like I've seen them at a favourite
haunt. If they don't look part of the furniture and they sort of start to run out
of the place . . . it's not his looks . . . I think it's things like just how comfort-
ably they walk, move, respond, whether they're like, um, bold or, um, or
whether they look a bit tentative.

Ian's account suggests he is savvy to the choreography of gay cruising and
negotiating anonymous sex. But it could also be read as evidence of how he
has come to embody the context that informs him.[40] That is to say, rather
than see him as moving in a context and as an effect of a context, similar
to Tim, we might recognize the informational context as embodied in him.
While both men could be argued to be products of a neo-liberal culture
"combining notions of informed consent, contractual interaction, free market choice, and responsibility in new ways,"[41] their articulation is informed
by work undertaken in and on their bodies by the viral load test and ARVs.
However, before I pursue this more coextensive account of a biomedically
informed person, I want to bring the question of risk and, hence, HIV more
directly into view.

In contrast to the contributions from Tim and Ian, the extract from
Andy below was initially obtained from a different study on risk understandings and practices.[43] Andy, as HIV-negative, had sought and com-
pleted a course of PEP, intended to prevent HIV infection after a suspected
exposure.[43] In the interview he was not asked the question of "How do you
feel about condoms?" as was used for those in the broader study. Rather,
he was asked what activity had led him to seek PEP. His commentary lends
itself to an analytic of "informed matter" but enables some development
of how the notion of *environment* or, in the language of prevention, *culture* might be rethought. According to the methodology of my previous
research I might have introduced his statement as offering a different perspective on risk, yet with some knowledge of HIV biotechnologies. But I
suggest that it offers considerably more than a different perspective on the
same phenomenon.

When you get to know someone . . . you start to take calculated risks . . . you say to yourself "X has trouble putting on a condom and keeping an erection . . . so as long as he pulls out." If you love someone then you take the risk . . . calculating the risk is trusting him and his zero viral load. I don't know what that [zero viral load] means where sperm count [viral load is measured in blood not seminal fluid] is concerned but it seems to me I've survived two encounters and not been infected. I think what was responsible for me not testing positive [after accidental ejaculation inside him] was X's zero viral load.

It would be easy to focus on Andy's explicit acknowledgment of his HIV-positive partner's "undetectable" viral load test result, reinterpreted to "zero viral load" and his relatively sophisticated grasp of HIV biomedicine that aligns him with the other interviewees cited here. But it is also important to consider how he is enacted as different in a number of key ways for prevention. He and his partner understand their intimacy in relation to their opposite HIV antibody status which carries the potential *for* infection to take place. Further, this is mediated by his partner's relation with ARVs as these intersect and affect the potential or, as he indicates, possible lack of potential for infection. In or *through* these relations with ARVs Andy, like the others cited here, is part of the making of a heterogeneous technologized field. It is not only that individuals within a culture come to embody the culture in ontologically different ways. That is to say, Andy is not only positioned differently within a context which he embodies. He embodies a context which is different from the others cited so far. While gay men may be understood to embody a now complex and heterogeneous informational context—as will become even more apparent in the next interview extract—they are also active in its making and its making as heterogeneous and multiple. To see prevention possibilities in this way is to give up what John Law and John Urry refer to as a "Euclidean reality of discrete entities of different sizes contained within discrete and very often homogeneous social spaces."[44] And while the benefits of this reconceptualization may be hard to decipher at this point, I conclude that it offers significant possibilities for methodological innovation in studies for prevention.

The final extract sheds a different light on the "risk calculus" evidently practiced by Tim and Ian. It also elaborates a context more potentially inclusive of Andy's position and HIV-negative status. In the words of Will, who is HIV-positive:

> Yeah, if I'm being receptive and it's a one-nighter and the condoms are there
> . . . I won't disclose my status, but I will leave it up to the other person who is
> being the active partner to put on a condom. . . . If they don't [use a condom]
> I figure well obviously they know the risk, the information is out there,
> boom. I also know the risk of them getting infected from me is very minimal.
> If on the other hand I'm being the active partner I'd always put a condom on,
> you know. I've had one instance where I didn't because I assumed he was
> HIV-positive because he didn't want to use a condom. He assumed I was HIV-
> negative because I didn't want to use a condom. Don't know how he figured
> that out, but that's where he was coming from. Two weeks down the track he
> found out I was positive and went for a test and it was the worst three months
> of my life. Worrying I'd infected him and merely because I hadn't commu-
> nicated before the incident. So we're both not having safe sex, but both for
> different reasons. So, I learnt from that. Obviously, it's better to talk than not
> talk because you can dig a hole for yourself if you don't. But, yeah, on the
> whole that's who I will stand as—if it's a one-nighter and they're going inside
> me, it's their responsibility for a condom. If I'm going inside someone else I'll
> always use a condom mainly for the guilt . . . I'd feel really bad if I ended up
> giving someone else HIV and they passed away from it and I'm still alive. I
> don't know how I'd mentally cope. So, maybe it's a preventative measure for
> my mental sanity that I use a condom as much as [for] safe sex.

Will offers insight into how HIV transmission may occur in what is mistakenly assumed as a shared informational context or, as Kippax and Race would
put this, his account shows how a "mismatch" can take place. As such, it provides a glimpse of the coming together of a diverse array of phenomena that
affect each other and that can also be argued are part of a dynamic heterogeneous assemblage. Will is equally aware of how the event—as he describes
it—contradicts the idea that knowledge is something that—as individuals—
we know in the same way. According to his account, his first assumption was
that in a context of safe sex campaigns on the importance of condoms, it is
reasonable to assume that anyone who doesn't request a condom before pene-
tration is HIV-positive.[45] But his account also demonstrates the possibility that

an HIV-negative man, in the seemingly same context of safe sex messages, may assume (perhaps involving some denial) that a positive man would—because he should—use a condom. A person who knows himself or herself as "without HIV" might (wrongly) assume that prevention begins at the locale of the virus. In fact Will's stated concern after the act, gives weight to this as he, as an HIV-positive man, has taken this on or *in*.[46] It is this taking in that helps constitute Will's reflexive consideration that the virus might be more damaging to a partner than it had, to date, been to himself.

From a prevention point of view, Will's after-the-act concern seems rather futile. Accepting that the logics put forward in the above extract are an indication of "mismatched strategies" and, hence, risk,[47] it is necessary to move beyond the question: Why are gay men, as a community, now significantly less homogeneous in their take-up of condoms than earlier in the epidemic? In place, we might ask: How can prevention strategies be developed, given the now apparent diversity in current "risk calculus"?

All four men cited here share the assumption that their partner's practice of UAI does not take place in ignorance. They also indicate a belief or chosen presumption that their sexual partner shares the same knowledge as themselves or, at least, sufficient knowledge to act against contracting HIV if he, the partner, chooses. The assumption is, no doubt, based on presence of safe sex messages in the form of posters, flyers, and advertisements beginning pre-ARVs, including those by McDiarmid. As I have mentioned above in discussion of Andy's experience, the differences evidenced in the men and most pronounced at the point that viral transmission might take place challenge the premises on which HIV prevention has been based, that is, that there is a homogeneous space that can continue to be enacted through prevention messages. Returning to Law and Urry's critique of Euclidean space and the presumption that discrete entities function within discrete and very often homogeneous social spaces, it may be helpful to rethink the space or, as some would say "culture" of prevention along the lines of Mike Michael's argument that a "'mutual warping' may take place between an 'entity' and 'its space.'" This enables space to be rethought as dynamic in its interrelatedness with what are more usually conceived as merely situated within it or passing through it.[48] Consequently, it becomes possible to conceive of the space or "culture" of HIV prevention as multiple and, moreover, the transformations that take place within it cannot be held or assumed to conform to its imagined static state. In the concluding section of this chapter, I consider some of the possibilities for prevention by rethinking the terrain in this way.

## CONCLUSION

This chapter commenced with reference to the decoupling of HIV and AIDS that took place with the use of ARVs and how, on the basis of this major change or watershed, the work of prevention has been changed. In order to put forward an argument for rethinking prevention, it has been necessary to review a set of presumptions about human agency. Throughout this chapter I have endeavored to convey that prevention involves a form of distributed agency and that the idea of gay men as "informed matter" or as historic entities—who are not only constitutive entities *of* their environment but contribute to the dynamic of the latter—provides a more complex and indeed richer field with which (not within which!) to intervene. Biotechnologies are evidently active in what it is to act as a gay man in relation to the virus and, going further afield, they may affect how any of us negotiate conditions for which biotechnologies are designed or have an identified relational affect. But as I have argued, they also have the capacity to partake in an altering of the properties of what it is to act. Tests, drugs, condoms, and epidemiological knowledge are already integral to those whose practices have become of paramount concern.

In order to respond to the current challenge or paradox of how to devise and utilize biomedical innovation to prevent and not enhance infection, it is worth pausing on the practice of UAI or anal intercourse without condoms as it has appeared throughout this chapter as "the marked" or non-normalized practice. That is, a sexual practice that incorporates condoms has become "the norm" despite what—prior to HIV prevention work—would have been regarded as not natural and therefore not normal. This remarkable reinvesting of what is regarded as "normal" practice—at least by significant numbers of gay men and public authorities supporting safe sex—apart from an otherwise assumed "natural" practice exemplifies the possibilities for reworking an historical and relational field.

The men cited above speak of themselves as part of a process that we might understand as reflective of a neo-liberal subject engaged in decisions of self that presume free choice and, with it, forms of consent based on some sort of limited contractual relationship.[49] But they can also be conceived as considerably more than this. Initially, Will's story and the apparent mismatch[50] may be read as taking place due to the coming together of two discrete bodies, informed by different knowledge and making different assumptions. But the story might also be understood as arising from an informational context that does not stop and start at the boundaries of these bodies, as if information or the traffic in information as flesh takes place only in the space between them. For the mismatch is embodied in, and making of, Will's and his partner's differences. Indeed, for Tim, Ian, Andy, Will, and Will's unnamed HIV-negative sex partner, the entity of HIV has varying meaning in the relational context of viral load tests, ARVs, and long-term self-knowledge of HIV-positive antibody status. And, to extend this argument, the relational context yields a different sort of personhood, heterogeneously informed—and not just discursively—through the historical route of living with HIV.

This different conception of *informed* embodied subjects requires a different sort of strategic thinking for prevention research and the development of prevention programs. Knee-jerk or even carefully deliberated responses fixed on the responsible or irresponsible human individual need to be replaced by more nuanced accounts of the relational process that biomedical interventions partake in and for which their design—involving a traffic in subject/body—can be held at least partially responsible. As I argued in chapter 3, biotechnologies need to meet and enhance the lives of those they claim to be designed for. In HIV prevention research this could translate into questions about how the virus has come to be a more fractured variable entity and in ways that challenge existing conceptions of choice. Or, for example, rather than focusing solely on the question of how gay men will behave if given the opportunity of PEP as briefly discussed in the introduction to this book and early on in this chapter, it could be more effective to ask what new material-semiotic assemblage will PEP or, indeed, other forms of intervention contribute to? If Dunbar's *Posithiv Sex Happens*—with its bodies connecting to each other and to an intravenous drip—challenged us to rethink the relational nature of medicine and illness, it might now be reread as a site of becoming, still reflective of the lives of those affected by HIV and more than ever underscoring the connectedness of biomedicine to sex in the dynamic space of the epidemic.

# 5

## THE HUMAN HOST: PERFORMATIVE
## AND RELATIONAL DIFFERENCE

it is not enough to claim that human subjects are constituted, for the construction of the human is a differential operation that produces the more and the less "human," the inhuman, the humanly unthinkable.

—Judith Butler, *Bodies That Matter: On The Discursive Limits of Sex*

Like nature, race has much to answer for; and the tab is still running for both categories.

—Donna J. Haraway, Modest_Witness@Second_Millennium:
FemaleMan@_MeetsOncoMouse™

for better biology . . .

WHAT DOES IT MEAN TO CLAIM THAT AIDS HAS A WOMAN'S FACE as Kofi Annan did while Secretary General of the United Nations? Or what might be concluded from various studies of pharmaceutical trials, including those for HIV, that find racial differences affect drug effectiveness? Such claims serve to highlight the significance of human difference in the field of illness and disease. With regard to HIV, they reflect a context in which there is growing attention to human host difference and a will to devise interventions more attuned to such. Indeed, it is apparent from the array of research studies now published in HIV specialist journals that human host difference has become a primary area of investigation for reducing infection rates as well as for devising more effective treatments and biomedical prevention such as vaccines. Yet, given what I have argued in the previous chapters of this book, it is necessary to ask whether the framing of such claims may impede their intended goal of better intervention. For they rely on a series of presuppositions. Most notably, there is the presumption of a stable distinction between "information" and "flesh" that prevents examination of a more intricate process in the materializing of HIV phenomena. Following the argument of Karen Barad, as one example of the critique I want to pursue here: To what extent are claims of gender and racial host differences materializations of a performative process that obscures its own role in the matter of difference? And further, if gender and racial differences were to be seen as effects of this process, what would this mean for devising interventions against HIV?

In the preceding chapters, I have claimed that technologies relied upon for deciphering the virus, drugs, and social and/or embodied subjects may be usefully understood as inevitably leaving their traces in what is more commonly presumed independent of, or external to, the work of such technologies. Another way of putting this is that the objects of our knowledge— for example HIV or the body—already embody the technology necessary to their representation and that recognizing this is critical to effective intervention.[1] Here, I turn this to claim that the categories of race and male/female difference perform difference in ways that come to be accepted as given, even while at the same time revealing a more heterogeneous and processual field. In contrast to standardized research conventions that are presumed to function in a highly constrained manner, that is, as if transparent modes of observation, I begin from the proposition that these conventions enact their object into being. I then consider some of the possible implications of this. Rather than view identity categories such as "race" or "gender" as stable entities, I argue that their ontological status be reconceived according to performative and relational conceptions of matter.

## SEX AND RACE ANEW IN THE HUMAN HOST OF HIV

Many national and international health and research initiatives now strive to deal more equitably with what they perceive as issues posed by social and biological human differences. According to Steven Epstein, in the United States this is the result of political campaigning, which has seen that tax dollars are no longer devoted to the health priorities of white males and that research is no longer based on the white Anglo male body as the norm.[2]

The focus is now directed toward "women"—a category of persons previously excluded from clinical trials—and persons referred to as members of either "racial" or "ethnic" groups, who are understood to be neglected in the delivery of health services.[3] However, as Epstein also notes, the intended meaning and usage of the categories is not at all clear, especially when it comes to translating them into medicine.[4] A Web site of the US National Institutes of Health (NIH) titled "NIH Policy on Reporting Race and Ethnicity Data: Subjects in Clinical Research" states:

> The Office of Management and Budget (OMB) defines minimum standards for maintaining, collecting and presenting data on race and ethnicity for all federal reporting agencies (including NIH). The categories in this classification are *social-political constructs and should not be interpreted as being anthropological in nature* [my emphasis]. The standards were revised in 1997 and now include two ethnic categories, "Hispanic or Latino" and "Not Hispanic or Latino." There are five racial categories: American Indian or Alaska Native; Asian; Black or African American; Native Hawaiian or Other Pacific Islander; and White. Reports of data on race and ethnicity shall use these categories. NIH is required to use these definitions to allow comparisons to other federal databases, especially the census and national health databases.[5]

The reference to categories as "social-political constructs" is, no doubt, intended to avoid a now well-refuted reduction of difference to biology that has enabled differentially designated notions of humanness. But the use of "ethnicity" along with "race" indicates the fraught nature of this terrain. If "ethnicity" is used to refer to differences recognized solely as social, with the direct intention of avoiding or refuting a biological source, then we might ask: what is intended in the use of "racial categories"? It is not difficult to assume from the above statement and as I shall show later in reference to HIV, that "ethnicity" and "race" are presumed in some way to be interchangeable and have important bearing on embodied health and illness. The slippage between "race" and "ethnicity" is paralleled by another slippage that can occasionally be observed when science uses the term "gender." Although the social sciences and humanities have asserted a nature/culture distinction and feminist approaches use the term 'gender' to emphasize that differences in capacities and opportunities are socially produced,[6] later it will be evident that the biological sciences do not always follow this usage.

Within the HIV field, a report from the primary US organization oriented to prevention and treatment of HIV, the US Centers for Disease Control and Prevention (CDC), titled "Inclusion of Women and Racial and Ethnic Minorities in Research" states in its opening paragraph:

> The Centers for Disease Control and Prevention is committed to protecting the health of *all* people regardless of their sex, race, ethnicity, national origin, religion, sexual orientation, socioeconomic status, or other characteristics. To the extent that participation in research offers direct benefits to the participants, under-representation of certain population subgroups denies them the opportunity to benefit. Moreover, for purposes of generalizing study results, investigators must include the widest possible range of population groups.[7]

It is apparent in the above statement that attention to the question of differences among humans in their relations with the virus—and irrespective of whether these differences are designated according to the terms of "sex," "gender," "race," "ethnicity," or other categories listed above—accords with the agenda of the NIH. It is also worth noting that this is not simply a reflection of funding criteria, although it is not difficult to make a case that the HIV field is highly affected by NIH funding.[8] The NIH requirement that race, ethnicity, and gender should be considered as factors in all forms of health and medical research dovetails with growing recognition of genetic variation across HIV human hosts. Both host genetic variation and gender factors—whether deemed social or biological—have become prominent objects in the HIV research field in the past ten years or so, as part of efforts to devise and implement more effective social and biomedical interventions. But given the murkiness of conceptions of human host difference, how does this work?

## DECIPHERING DIFFERENCE

Without specifying why race-based categories are now in frequent use for deciphering genetic variation in the HIV human host, among the most cutting edge and sophisticated areas of biogenetics, the categories are emerging as a means of tailoring more effective HIV treatment and prevention. As I discuss in some detail in the later sections of this chapter referring to specific scientific research studies, there are now numerous clinical trials taking place across the globe that are expressly designed to (1) involve people from self-identified racial and ethnic backgrounds; and/or (2) form comparative studies to establish the extent that racial/ethnic differences (the categories are often collapsed) may be significant in disease progression and drug interventions; and following from this, in some instances (3) utilize the establishment of racial and ethnic differences to point to the work of host genetics in immunological susceptibility to or protection against the virus.

Although likely to be seen as significantly, if not wholly, different from the practice of eugenics, the social, political, ethical, but also medical implications of this usage of "race," "racial," or "ethnic" categories remain relatively unexplored. We might deduce that the broad field of HIV advocacy and social inquiry is either unaware of the emergence of racial typing in science and/or not equipped to engage with the type of questioning this now necessitates. This is even though earlier work showed how racist conflations of Africa with sex and disease contributed to the spread of the epidemic.[9] Certainly within the area of science where the category appears, there is little query about what is assumed by race or ethnicity when the two are used interchangeably to refer to genetic difference.

Indicative of a presumptiveness about race, none of the studies that I have so far come across in my own preliminary research efforts has provided any explanation of the criteria used to racially identify research participants. Indeed, it is only through informal inquiries that I have learned that self-identification is a basis for recruitment in countries such as the UK or US. When clinical trials are conducted in countries where a region is assumed to consist of a culturally self-identified stable population, race is taken as self-evident; for example, a clinical trial in a region in North India will involve individuals from the same racial group.

In light of the ambiguous use of racial identifiers, it could be argued that medical interventions developed from studies reliant on such identifiers will not succeed at least not as anticipated. Further, if Butler's claim is right: that the construction of the human is inevitably a differential operation, then it is likely that such studies may enable normative and exclusionary forms of discrimination.[10]

Alongside the development of new biogenetic technologies aimed at establishing a more precise knowledge of how the virus gains entry to the human cell, how host factors may affect infectivity, and how viral progression in vivo comes to differ across individuals, there has also been an increase in epidemiological studies that shed light on why some groups fare worse than others in relation to HIV infection. Kofi Annan's dramatic claim that "AIDS has a woman's face" puts on notice the urgent need to address phenomena specific to the increase in infected women.[11] However, Annan's statement was coined to underscore not just numbers but a complex array of factors that are now understood to contribute to the greater vulnerability of women to HIV/AIDS. Central among these factors is women's reliance on men's use of the male condom. Some critics argue that the absence of a technology able to be implemented directly by women is powerful evidence of how HIV interventions are dominated by a male-centered approach, based on a conception of the male body and operating in the interests of it.[12] Indeed, it seems that the gendered nature of sexual relations translates directly into higher numbers of infections in women.

Yet despite the weight and importance of a gender analysis for mobilizing research agendas including those for vaginal and anal microbicides (more than twenty-five years after identification of the virus as sexually transmitted),[13] the emphasis on women's vulnerability and the notion of a male-centered or masculinist approach tend to imply—as I later argue in relation to the problem of gender or sex difference in clinical research—that there is a binary and that only one side of it is recognized. That is to say, the claim of male-centrism fails to recognize its own normative function, along with the normative function of the binary itself. Critiques that rest on a notion of gender difference offer little for addressing what I want to argue is a more insidious process of materialization. There is need for a conception of embodied difference that goes beyond an imagined terrain of stable self-identical units or bodies of matter.

My inference that "gender" or the "gendered nature of the epidemic" requires interrogation should not be understood to deny the presence of phenomena that have lead to such conceptual usage or framing. For example, it should not be taken to deny what is understood as risk linked to genital physiology and which, in epidemiological terms, shows that male-to-female transmissibility is about twice that of female-to-male transmission.[14] Nor should it be assumed to deny phenomena that have been reduced to a concept of gendered power relations.[15] Rather, the need to question the deployment of gender as a concept follows from its static and contradictory framing that delimits other potentially more effective accounts. While I do not want to elide male/female difference or differences that can be identified between one population and another, new modes for conceptualizing this are imperative. HIV does not affect all bodies in the same way. Or, to turn this slightly given the new emphasis on the human host and to make a little more of the latter's palpability, all bodies do not engage with HIV in the same way. Yet, despite the abundance of data now available from molecular scientific studies and epidemiological social scientific studies, there is little clarity on how to conceive these entities of body and virus as they are recognized to cohere in a life-threatening relationship.

## MATERIALIZING RACE

Through a review of some recent HIV clinical trials, I want to begin to examine some of the means by which science materializes and dematerializes the substance of its inquiries. It is because of the already established contentiousness of "race" and, to a lesser extent, "ethnicity" that I begin with studies focused on these designations, followed by those that feature a binary of male/female sex/gender in the assessment of difference. Those selected illustrate the confusion and slippage that occur when trying to establish medical phenomena through a reliance on categories. They also evidence the way that a pre-identified categorization may be materialized or made more concrete through conventional research practice.

### Case Study One: Reiterations of Race across Difference

In the paper "Influence of CCR5 Promoter Haplotypes on AIDS Progression in African-Americans," Ping An and coauthors report on findings from a study that (to paraphrase a little) hypothesized that CCR5 promoter variants—features on human host immune cells—in HIV-1-infected African Americans affect the rate of progression to AIDS. To put this more simply, An and colleagues investigated whether a specific immune system genetic characteristic (within the human host and to which the term haplotypes refers) affects the progression to AIDS. The study was based on previous data that had shown that two CCR5 variants accelerate AIDS progression in Caucasians. Without explanation of what constitutes "race" as a research variable—African Americans or Caucasians—the paper concludes:

> Unlike the CCR5-^32 mutation which is found only in people of northern European descent, the CCR5P1 allele [gene location] has frequencies greater than 40% in Caucasians, Asians and people of African descent, thus the CCR5P1 allele may have a more general effect on AIDS pathogenesis worldwide. The identification of additional functional polymorphisms [more genetic diversity] among ethnic/racial groups may provide valuable insights into differences observed in transmission and pathogenesis of HIV-1 globally.[16]

When this statement is put alongside those in a later paper "Patterns of Ethnic Diversity among the Genes That Influence AIDS" first authored by Cheryl Winkler and that includes many of the authors from the An Ping study, it is clear that 'ethnic/racial groups' is based on an evolutionary model of human difference. There is discussion on how human diversity is the result of migratory patterns, including the forced removal of people from western Africa to European-founded colonies, and through pressure from deadly infectious agents and regional environmental factors. Presumably Winkler and colleagues' evolutionary theory has led them to assume the appropriateness of using the categories "Caucasians," "Asians," and "people of African descent." But it is also apparent that diversity at the level of the human genome has already been assumed to produce stable categories of persons, and the main work is to provide an explanation for the form this may take. That is to say, the categories are assumed as given and an explanation is provided for their evolution. Consistent with studies in the field more generally, the An and colleagues' paper does not explain how the individual trial participants were assigned to race categories. But it is the conclusion to the team's second paper that is especially problematic. Offering an evolutionary prediction, the authors state:

> the current HIV-1/AIDS epidemic may soon deposit its own footprints in human genomes in the form of rapidly expanding protective haplotypes and selective sweeps of advantageous alleles.[17]

The statement reflects not simply the authors' evolutionary theory of how we have come to be fleshed as a series of genetically different groups but, also, how this theory leads them to imagine human-ness according to a conceptual framework that makes no allowance for the inherence of technology in our being, even after having acknowledged a phenomenon such as migratory patterns.[18] That is, they imagine humans as isolated yet affected; apart or distinct from forces other than the coming together of viral and human genetics. Indeed, human genetics emerge through a performative of race and purely so. Contributory factors, namely asymmetrical health infrastructure and treatment access, are excluded. Although it is important to recognize evidence that suggests that some individuals may be genetically immune to the virus due to a variation in their CD4 cell structure that disinhibits viral entry, this variation is unlikely to make a significant difference to the survival of a population.[19] It is far more likely that the intricacies of economically and politically mediated pharmaceutical intervention will have more of an effect on who survives and who may or may not reproduce without passing on the virus.

Before moving on to discuss the presumption of identity categories and their force in materializing pre-given sex and/or gender divisions, I will provide one further example of how race, or its sometimes stand-in "ethnicity" as a sign of difference, is used as a research variable in a highly convincing way. In the course of doing so, I want to introduce a notion of relationality.[20] Consistent with the overall project of this book, I want to lay the ground for engaging with difference in a way that is not encumbered by a nature/culture or information/flesh split and presumptions of representation that follow from these distinctions. But I also want to offer something towards materially effective intervention and this is a point, as I have suggested in chapter 2, that requires a departure from the conception of performativity provided by Butler.

"Validity of Existing CD4+ Classification in North Indians, in Predicting Immune Status," by V. Satya Suresh Attili and colleagues, offers evidence to support the establishment of a different case definition of HIV for North Indian HIV patients in comparison with a "western case definition."[21] The study followed others that had found "ethnic" variability in the CD4 lymphocyte count. The authors state that "in general, Caucasians have higher CD4 counts than Asians. Among Africans, some populations have higher

CD4 counts than Caucasians while others have lower CD4 counts." An important stated outcome of this reported diversity is the possibility that non-Caucasians, who have lower CD4 cell levels, are less likely to progress to AIDS than their Caucasian counterparts. Indeed, the study by Attili and colleagues found "the mean CD4 count among normal [people without HIV] North Indians is significantly lower than that in the western population and parallels that of the Chinese." While a longitudinal study is noted as necessary before guidelines can be drawn up in response to this difference, it is apparent that the category "North Indians" was relatively self-evident for the researchers. Indeed, they state that North Indians "constitute a distinct group among the populations of the India subcontinent."[22] When put alongside other studies, the findings from Atilli's study may yield important clinical benefits. The inferred difference between the categories may also contribute to research on host genetics. In the context of this discussion, however, I want to argue that—similar to the CCR5 study—by comparing pre-identified racial groups, for example, Chinese and Caucasians, the study has effectively materialized a version of "race." It has materialized a statistically significant difference that accords with pre-identified genetically inferred categories and, in doing so, performs these categories as real.

## Performative Relational Ontologies

From the above studies aimed at contributing to urgently needed treatment and prevention developments, it is possible to see that racial categories have altered significantly in meaning and consequent status since their usage in the late nineteenth and early to mid-twentieth centuries. Nevertheless, at least outside the HIV research field, their usage remains contentious and, more important, the question of how to deal with this tension in light of the need for better interventions remains.

In the essay "Standards, Populations, and Difference," Fraser summarizes some of the current debate on race as it has centered on claims by Risch, Burchard, Ziv Elad, and Tang in their paper "Categorization of Humans in Biomedical Research: Genes, Race and Disease." The team claims the validity of using racial categories as genetic indicators on the basis of geo-historical factors. Fraser brings special clarity to their argument and offers new insight into how we might understand race through statistical data on genetic correlations. She states that "race," as Risch and colleagues discuss it, "is not the bare existence of a race gene that causes things (diseases, specific responses to therapeutic interventions) but rather, in a more attenuated and indirect model of causality, the processes that give rise to populations of actual bodies."[23] The term "actual bodies," taken from A. N. Whitehead, is important here as it refers to everything that has enabled the performative achievement of race. It can be equated with "actual entities" of which Whitehead states:

> "Actual entities"—also termed "actual occasions"—are the final real things of which the world is made up. There is no going behind actual entities to find anything more real. They differ among themselves. God is an actual entity, and so is the most trivial puff of existence in far off empty space. But though there are gradations of importance, and diversities of function, yet in the principles which actuality exemplifies all are on the same level . . . actual entities are drops of experience, complex and interdependent."[24]

There is, then, no settling or lapsing into an either/or of "biology" versus "social construction" and there is not an occlusion of process of knowing in the Risch et al. study. According to Fraser, for Risch and colleagues, there is no "clear conception of race outside of statistics." Statistics are part of the material performativity of race. They are part of its becoming. Indeed, to the extent that "race" endures—and in ways that are more widely contested than other achievements such as sex difference or humanness—it may be understood as an assemblage in process and open to interrogation.

Drawing on the work of Manuel Delanda and his Deleuzian conception of "state space"—a term intended to characterize the processual relationality of "actual entities"—Fraser says "bodies and physical spaces are inextricably conjoined, reorganizing, and reproblematizing themselves "as the assemblage stabilizes itself through the mutual accommodation of its heterogeneous elements."[25] Such heterogeneous elements are difficult to untangle and are themselves abstractions in the sense that they are products of technologies of knowledge and inevitable as such. In other words, what we have in "race" is a contingent processual entity that encompasses what might ordinarily be presumed divided or incumbent on a nature/culture bifurcation. The notion of an assemblage enables a more temporal and spatial consideration of the emergence of difference and, in doing so, makes possible a more dynamic conception of matter as a real yet *in transformation* performative and relational effect.

At this point I want to pause on my reintroducing the phrase "performative effect." For throughout this chapter I have been developing two parallel lines of approach to the question of matter. While I do not wish to spend too much time on identifying where they might be argued to differ as well as concur, it may be helpful to clarify the purpose of engaging with a Foucault/Butler/Barad and a Whitehead/Deleuze/Barry/Fraser approach. Fraser makes clear that the actual entity is the effect of value enfolded into matter.[26] This is leveled against the presupposition of the natural sciences that values can be ruled out. There is an emphasis here on an ontology that is the effect of a dynamic process and one that includes the observing apparatus. Importantly, while a Butlerian performativity might be understood to shy away from any ontological claim, Butler's work may still be understood as a reformulation of the ontological <u>and</u> with direct emphasis on the role of power in its materialization. To reiterate, Butler claims that matter is the effect of the coextensive nature of investiture and materiality.[27] Hence, investiture can be understood as equivalent in meaning to value in the sense that objects or entities do not emerge without it. However, when used in Whitehead's sense, value may also be understood as more contingent. In other words, the emphasis on relationality suggests value is as much part of the association as other contributing forces, that is, it emerges through the association.[28]

In chapter 2, I argued that an extended account of the generative effects of intervention is necessary on the part of science and social science and, in chapter 3, I suggested that a network or relational analytic must also consider asymmetrical forces in the process. A similar claim can be made about the notion of population difference in its relation to biomedicine and biotechnologies. For however the identified genetic or embodied ethnic differences are claimed, these cannot be distinguished in any absolute sense from the technologies enabling their identification.

## Case Study Two: Binary Difference

"[S]ex" is a regulatory ideal whose materialization is compelled, and this materialization takes place (or fails to take place) through certain highly regulated practices. In other words, "sex" is an ideal construct which is forcibly materialized through time. . . . That this reiteration is necessary is a sign that materialization is never quite complete, that bodies never quite comply with the norms by which their materialization is impelled.[29]

For most people working across the sciences male/female difference, the binary of sex, is an originary and continuing unchanged essence of human life. For instance, Burchard and colleagues treat male/female difference as a "biologic category," whereas "racial and ethnic categories are said to arise primarily through geographic, social and cultural forces and, as such, are not stagnant, but potentially fluid."[30] Yet although scientific data, as I illustrate below, presumes the notion of two distinct and, to some extent, selfsame/stable homogeneous male and female entities, its empirical complexity contests this.

I begin with a study by Sterling and colleagues titled "Initial Plasma HIV-1 RNA Levels and Progression to AIDS in Women and Men" that assessed whether viral load measures in women provide the same surrogate marker of disease progression as they do in men. Its conclusion:

Although the initial level of HIV-1 RNA [viral load] was lower in women than in men, the rates of progression to AIDS were similar. Treatment guidelines that are based on the viral load [measures of viral particles in an individual's sample of blood], rather than the CD4+ lymphocyte count [human immune cells also assessed from an individual blood sample], will lead to differences in eligibility for antiretroviral treatment according to sex. [31]

In the previous section of this chapter on race and ethnicity, variation in viral load measures was raised in relation to the ethnic differences between "Caucasians" and "North Indians" and "Chinese." Sex difference here confirms the problem of "the universal body" that has served as a model for the natural sciences and, like the material discussed earlier, paradoxically appears to affirm the necessity of recognizing bodily difference as set out in the NIH charter. Indeed, the above study lends weight to arguments for more knowledge of host genetic variation. Before considering what to make of this, I want to outline two further studies that engage, in varying ways, the categories of male and female.

As mentioned earlier, epidemiological data has established that women, as a category, are more likely to become infected from a positive male partner through vaginal intercourse than the category of men when having vaginal intercourse with a positive female partner.[32] Although I initially raised this in reference to greater female physiological susceptibility to HIV—attributed to the design of female anatomy—a recent study by Coombs and colleagues suggests that at least part of the explanation may be due to men being more infectious than women. The suggestion is based on the finding that men more frequently have detectable HIV in their sexual fluids than women.[33] The data does not detract from female anatomical susceptibility, but it does imply that a more relational conception of HIV infection may be important.

Similar to the study by Atilli, a study by the CASCADE Collaboration titled "Differences in CD4 Cell Counts at Seroconversion and Decline among 5739 HIV-1-Infected Individuals with Well-Estimated Dates of Seroconversion" used diagnostic measures as a marker and materializer of difference, although in reference to sex difference. The study, which involved what are regarded as large numbers due to the combining of data from a number of studies, found that although women and men have different levels of CD4 cells at the time of seroconversion the rate of decline is the same for both.[34] The study also found that "subjects infected through sex between men and women" had, on average, a less steep CD4 decline than the rest of the subjects (those infected through injecting drug use or through sex between men). The authors' note that "the biologic reason as well as the clinical relevance of the differences in immunologic response by exposure category observed in this study remains unclear," and suggest that

"female sex hormones possibly affecting CD4 levels may provide one explanation and that the data on gay men and male IDUs—which is noted to contradict other studies which have found that *all* men have lower CD4 counts than women at the time of seroconversion—may be due to lifestyle factors of gay men and male IDUs (for example, use of drugs or constant immune activation due to STIs)."[35]

In summary, the study could be used to highlight the need for more categories. But it could also be argued that its findings demonstrate the need for a conceptual approach able to deal with its enactment of categories of difference. Put another way, what is required is an approach able to consider a complex mix of historically constituted factors, including the research design and research presuppositions in this.

Further supporting the need for a more relational conception are findings from a study by Gray and colleagues, titled "Pregnancy and the Risk of Incident HIV in Rakai, Uganda, a Cause for Concern" that found women may be more vulnerable to HIV infection when they are pregnant. According to the findings, pregnant women have an infection rate more than double that among other women. Having ruled out what it refers to as possible cultural explanations for the doubling of HIV incidence in pregnant women, the authors suggest that the cause may lie with hormonal factors affecting changes at a cellular level where the virus gains entry or creates changes to the immune system induced by the presence of a fetus.[36] When combined with the above studies, the finding of differences between infected groups and, most notably, *within* the category "female" confirms the inadequacy of not only the universal male body, which the NIH appears to be attempting to overcome, but the inadequacy also of relying on and comparing categories as if they bear some inherent stability. Without suggesting that pre-identified variables can be avoided, on the basis of the above studies, host differences could be usefully conceptualized here—as I have begun to suggest of racially identified host difference—as an assemblage of enfolding matter, including the performative work of the category "female." For Gray and colleagues' findings are not simply about factors that reside within the pregnant female but, rather, findings that emerge through the category of the "the pregnant female" in the context of the study design.

## CONFUSING CATEGORIES

I now want to situate the categories of male/female in a manner that overlaps and further complicates what has been suggested of the category of "race." In particular, I want to take up one of the impetuses for considering the above-cited studies together and pursue the question of whether there is something that the two distinct areas of categorization—race and male/female—can learn from each other. That is to say, what can the binary of male/female difference draw from the resurfaced race/ethnicity category? Is the binary of sex difference grounded in biology or is it an effect of the informational context, a gender performative? Is race difference both an ideological construct and an indicator of genetic difference? Alternatively and following the findings of medical science discussed below, can or should we even assume that individual genetic identity is the essential aspect of our natural being? Finally, how might the use of any category be evaluated in medical phenomena?

In specific reference to studies inclusive of, but extending beyond, the HIV field, Epstein notes how the notion of "gender" moves across a nature/culture or biological/social divide in ways that presume but also muddle the notion of a given biologic substrata:

> [C]onfusion about the relation between the biological and the social has the effect of destabilising consensus about the drawing of generalisations within and across the sex/gender divide. At the same time, health professionals and researchers are likely to resolve such confusion by falling back on reduction-ist assumptions: firstly, that socially salient markers of difference, such as sex/gender, are invariably the ones that matter most in medicine; and second, that medical differences between men and women, once discovered, require no further explanation, because they simply reflect the fact that men and women are biologically different.[37]

Although male and female bodily grounded difference is unlikely to be questioned even if its basis is not always clear, there is ample evidence to contest this conception of difference. Within the areas of queer theory, sexuality, and gender studies, the binary of sexual difference has been exposed as not simply normative but cutting into—in a most literal manner—the very matter of what a body can or cannot be. According to Cheryl Chase, in her essay "Hermaphrodites with Attitude: Mapping the Emergence of Intersex Political Activism,"[38] one in a hundred births involve babies whose sex at birth is not clearly assignable to the distinct categories of male or female and, like herself, most are then subject to medical correction. While the numbers may come as a surprise for some, the intervention of medicine may not. Or, to qualify, medical intervention to assign "biologic" sex identity to one or the other side of the binary may not come as a surprise until it is consciously recorded that this is likely to involve removal of reproductive organs, including genitalia. To conform to an external conception of a two-body model, many individuals are corrected in ways that diminish their bodily capacities. Intersex, in medical terms, does not, in itself, pose a threat to the viability of the body. In many cases the arguments for a cultural or at least collaborative "biologic" making of the sexed body prevail, for instance in Chase's case where her capacities for genital organ-associated orgasm and for reproduction were removed in order to locate her on one side of the binary. Despite the presumption that our systems of understanding follow from nature, it seems that we can only know nature according to the terms of our technologies for doing so. Chase refers to "herself" because she has been "corrected" to perform so according to language. To assume a speaking position, moreover, to be present is already to be one of the two pronouns.

A further challenge to humanness, and not only to the two-body model but to the self-same individual genetic bodily identity imagined in this model, is posed by bodies identified as chimeras or mosaics. The definition of a chimera is that it incorporates two sets of genes that may be variably distributed through the body.[39] For instance, hair or ovaries may be of a genetic identity different from the kidney.[40] Relevant here is that the above phenomenon may pass entirely unnoticed unless genetic testing of different parts of the body is carried out. Recently, two cases of women, both of whom had conceived and given birth to their children, received media coverage when it was found that their genetic identities showed they could not in fact, or in conventional "common" sense, be the natural mothers of their offspring. Indeed, in biologic-genetic terms they are not the mothers of their children. The phenomenon provokes question of what it is that we presume when we call on the notion of hereditary genetic essence or, more simply, a homogeneous identity.

## NORMS, INVESTITURE OR ENFOLDINGS

The theories of performativity, as well as attention to relationality and assemblages, offer a way of situating phenomena in the field of HIV as entities of change. This is important for recognizing the mutually affective nature of intervention and its targeted phenomena. According to Bruno Latour, it is imperative that affective relations are recognized as the crux of what might be conceived as human life and that their dynamic nature must necessarily involve a maximizing and multiplying of difference. Indeed, the conception of difference is a feature of human life. However, Latour's conception of this difference is not as a conventional biological scientist might see it. That is, it is not difference to be identified by technology. Rather, it is difference elicited in relation to technology. Latour argues that the maximizing or eliciting of differences through a collaborative process of technology and what appears as human substance is important to better science. Given the pervasive nature of the norm as evidenced in the treatment of sexed bodies and even the notion of individual genetic essence (does an individual stop being so if they have two sets of genes?), Latour's alternative methodology is of special interest.[41] He asks: "Under what conditions can we mobilize the body in our speech in such a way that we are not immediately led to the usual discussions about dualism and holism?"[42] He follows with an argument on affective relationality, using as his example the perfume kit or *maletter à odeurs* for training people to detect different scents. In reference to the acquiring of sensitivity to different scents, he states: "The teacher, the kit and the session are what allow differences in the odours to make the trainees do something different every time . . . ." The observation of a new capacity implies a transforming entity, the specific and varied becoming of an entity. In this way, Latour casts the body as always engaged in—as part of its becoming—ongoing or processual differences achieved through human instruction and non-human technologies. It is by attending to these emergent differences, or "body talk," that it becomes possible to conceptualize a dynamic relational entity.

Although I have reservations about the applicability of the unqualified celebration of the generation of differences in the context of the perfume industry to the field of HIV, Latour offers a valuable example of a performative and relational process. It can be modified, in reference to HIV, to distinguish between affective differences, that is, between differences that need to be maximized against or in place of others destructive of the body.

## CONCLUSION

Throughout the epidemic the categories of human difference have been fodder for the intensification of stigmatization and discrimination, with death-inducing effects. Taking an optimistic view, it could be that the type of studies outlined above will move beyond contemporary categories as we currently know them and possibly bearing in mind the evident performative and relational nature of "nature," whether this is, for example, the human host, the virus, modes of infectivity, or viral load measures. Differences might multiply to the extent that race and even sex categorizations will be undermined as they prove too crude a guide for research or clinical practice. However, it is also possible that new ways of locating difference will continue to conform to an existing and long-standing regime where humanness is differentially measured. Either way, it will be necessary to monitor closely, as Rabinow says, the work of culture in the making of flesh but, equally, how flesh is a critical feature of information.

The generating of difference through studies that claim to merely identify difference may partake in the long history of differential ways of valuing. Yet this activity could also bear the potential for undermining what Joan Scott has referred to as "the prototypical human individual," which reflects and instates a normative intelligibility.[43] While in some instances it may be useful, even necessary, to work with a proposed norm or, indeed, category of identity—bearing in mind its propositional nature—this chapter has emphasized the need and possibilities of recognizing that it, the (normative) object of inquiry, is an achievement of a performative and relational process. By making apparent a radically different ontology, I have highlighted a potential in the interrogation of categories and, here, especially in reference to the results of clinical trials. For besides arguing for a mode of reflexiveness similar to what I have argued for in chapter 2, it is also possible that the increasing array of data—arising through scientific study—is a rich source of challenge to current presumptions of HIV host identity.

# 6

## CONCLUSION

I think maybe I might go and find I don't have it [HIV] because how come my viral load is undetectable? It used to be medium and now they [doctors] say it is "undetectable." I often ask myself should I go to another clinic and have another [HIV antibody] test there. Because I feel it might be negative.

THE VIRAL LOAD TEST HAS BEEN AN IMPORTANT SOURCE OF INQUIRY throughout this book, and recalling the above statement by a woman I interviewed some years ago, here named Leila, seems an especially poignant way to conclude. The statement was made in the context of a discussion about her experience of living with HIV and how—having come to the UK from Zimbabwe and when, on becoming ill, an HIV antibody test confirmed a diagnosis of AIDS—she had been put on ARVs and had "recovered" her health. That is to say, the statement could be read as indicating some confusion about the meaning of an antibody test result because of its ready linking with her initial visible/experiential HIV infection. But to see her query as such would be to miss the performative function of the information/flesh distinction and its curious contrary fixing of a dynamic according to which interventions are then designed. Although for those in the medical field there will be no doubt about Leila's HIV antibody positive status *and* continued infection with HIV, her conjecture is based on empirical grounds that it is the presence of the virus—with its potential or apparent deleterious effects on the body (most notably on immune system cells) and communicable possibility—that is the real concern for those who are found to carry HIV antibodies.[1] Her conjecture captures much of what I have sought to convey throughout this book, signaled by the phrase, "a traffic in information as flesh." I take her statement not simply as about a test reading of virus but about the work of a biomedical test.

Leila's query can be readily understood as: What does it mean to be HIV antibody positive if the virus is not apparent? How does it matter that a person may carry antibodies to the virus, if the virus itself—the destructive force—is not only "undetectable" but not developing into AIDS? I draw these questions in particular because they foreground two interlinked themes of this book—information as flesh and the work of intervention—and reiterate the need for concepts akin to the dynamic nature of "nature." Tests to detect antibodies to HIV or HIV viral particles have featured in almost every chapter and always with some reference to their performative function. Despite their enactment as mere observational or diagnostic devices presumed to provide transparent access to their object, inevitably such tests come to be embedded in the materialization of their object. What allows a test to be viewed as a mere observational device is the presumption that information and flesh are distinct. For the bifurcation of "information *and* flesh" or "sign *and* materiality" obscures the performative process. And this, I have argued, hinders the potential for a more reflexive and refined (or redefined) approach to intervention. By holding fast to the bifurcation, it is difficult—perhaps nearly impossible—to perceive the generative force of our interventions and, critically, how this force might be intercepted in novel ways. From Leila's query and the suggestion that another clinic might re-test her antibody status to find she is no longer "HIV-positive," we might deduce that sign or information alone—in this account, antibody *status*—has little or at least a different meaning if siphoned off from the real (detectable virus) fleshed entity. Of course, and as I have already indicated, according to current medical understanding, "undetectable" does not mean not present. And while Leila is quite possibly aware of this, she remains, not surprisingly, sceptical of the reading of her result as it does not sufficiently comply or, to be more succinct, appears as information but without flesh.

## AGENCY AND ETHICS

The point of orientation for my own queries of HIV has been the decoupling of HIV from AIDS with the introduction of ARVs. More than twelve years since the establishment of ARVs as effective for suppressing viral replication, it is apparent that what once seemed like a pharmacological triumph has had profound effects. While most of those requiring treatment still await the arrival or feasible implementation of the drugs, I have posed ARVs as an unsatisfactory privilege. Bizarre as it may seem to put these words together, I hope the double entendre conveys my view that their partnering requires something more of intervention.

As I wrote this conclusion I searched Cindy Patton's book *Globalizing AIDS* for guidance on how to approach the transformations that have and continue to occur with an ongoing epidemic.[2] What I found was a sense of unspeakable loss. The loss of those who died in the earlier stage of the epidemic in the United States and the ongoing loss that endures. And while I do not want to claim that I have sufficiently grasped the sentiments that inform the work of someone who has been so formative in my own work, the despair that any of us might experience about an epidemic that can be claimed "the most scrutinised and studied and analysed disease in the history of medicine"[3] provokes me to take up another double theme—agency and ethics—that began this book and that features in a number of sections.

Across the broad-ranging field of inquiry concerned with HIV and AIDS, engagement with notions of agency and ethics remains restricted to a conception of an individual who may or may not act appropriately toward himself or herself and others or, else, to groups of individuals involved in conducting research with human subjects. That is to say, concepts of agency and ethics are not applied to the pressing questions: How is it that millions continue to die from AIDS? How is the remedy for HIV infection so seemingly complex that the previous question is possible? According to what modes of knowing has the virus entered into the disciplinary domains of the sciences, social sciences, and humanities? How is it enacted in the space of the clinic or the treatment information pamphlet or the clinical trial? Yet, according to the performative approach I have utilized in my discussions, agency may be queried in relation to all of the above and in a manner that shows it extends as a force for action and effect well beyond that of an active individual or group of individuals. It would be difficult to locate a single or originary source to which the effects of the epidemic may be traced. However, this does not mean there is no accountability and, hence, the question of ethics should not be lost here. A distributed notion of agency does not exclude questions of right or wrong and, associated with these, questions then of responsibility. Rather, as it allows for the work of non-human contributors in the materialization of wanted and unwanted effects, it foregrounds other areas where our work may be ethically accountable and makes more apparent the work of design—diagnostic, pharmaceutical, condom, pill shape and number, textual expression, clinical trials. The list goes on.

As agency is conceived as a dynamic and relational force, ethics shift from normative notions of right and wrong to an emergent property in what is wanted or not. It becomes inherent to the questions above and to Leila's also. As each question opens onto others, it becomes possible to begin to query an increasing specificity taking place from the global to the most micro. For instance, as Race states in chapter 2, and as alluded to by Leila's query as well, the micro active viral load test does more than provide the basis for pharmacological management of HIV.[4] It is active in what Nikolas Rose and Carlos Novas have termed is a somatic individual, birthed through new molecular knowledges and with whom comes a new source of relations to self and others.[5] As it reconfigures what it means to be HIV-positive, it delivers new possibilities, new choices, and with these new obligations. For Leila, like millions of others, "undetectable" does not free her from having to take ARVs. It is likely to mean the prospect of her life is extended and without doubt this is of critical importance. But, paradoxically, the freeing up may involve her in negotiating the possibility of transmitting the infection to an intimate sexual other or to offspring during pregnancy and labor.[6] On a continued everyday basis, it may involve dealing with the toxic effects or fear of such from ARVs. Plus there may be the avoiding of disclosure of her HIV status that comes with strict dosing adherence and remains a possible individual concern, even after thirty years of the epidemic.

Within the extended account of agency and ethics that I am proposing is a conception of technology as that which makes our being or becoming possible and, conversely, how we manage or perform this forms part of the ethical terrain. Perhaps one of the most founding paradoxes of our thought is Martin Heidegger's claim that we can only distinguish our original involvement with technology by conceptually elevating and separating out "human-ness" from what is always invariably there within and of us. The point is repeated by Latour when he says: "there is no sense in which humans may be said to exist as humans without entering into commerce with what authorizes and enables them to exist (i.e., to act)."[7] Hence, as ethics is inherent to the work of increasingly technologized interventions in the molecular gaze of biomedicine, ethics may also be understood as present in the move to challenge the seemingly self-evident unsatisfactory privilege of ARVs.

## ONTOLOGICAL POLITICS

At its simplest, the methodological approach I have undertaken has been directed toward unravelling some of the most rigid premises of the epidemic. However, the strategy has not precluded the enactment of more phenomena. Law and Urry note:

> social inquiry and its methods are productive: they [help to] make social realities and social worlds. They do not simply describe the world as it is, but also enact it . . . [and] if social investigation makes worlds, then it can, in some measure, think about the worlds it wants to help to make. It gets involved, in other words, in the business of "ontological politics."[8]

Unlike conventional scientific and social scientific approaches within the HIV field, the key premise of this book has been that a challenge to the distinction between information *and* flesh will enable more insight into the work we do and generate. But this has also raised new questions about how to think about their relation or the traffic taking place in their enactment in ways that may offer better purchase on the object of inquiry. Throughout this book, the term traffic has conveyed a productive or constitutive activity—and not necessarily a happy one—that involves a transfer of sorts taking place. Whether it be understood as a vehicle for following the dynamic relationality between nature and culture or information and flesh or simply to convey movement in what are often presumed as fixed, non-relational entities, it has been intended to de-naturalize but not erase entirely such distinctions. The distinctions we make between a realm of signs and that of materiality—metaphysical absence and presence—are not a problem in themselves. Rather it is the work they perform. As Lury in particular shows, there is a danger in their refuting as distinct, for a crucial life difference may be erased.[9] Lury's contribution is a reminder that there is a history embedded in matter and it is critical that we do not lose sight of this. To do so would, in effect, re-*naturalize* by abstracting out the agency and ethics inherent to materialization or the matter of matter, which I am keen to foreground in this final section. Any effective intervention must establish a relation of sorts with what is already assumed apparent, and throughout this book I have argued that this requires attention to the performative and relational nature of appearance. In sum, it could be said that the project of this book has been to open up the conceptual and, by implication, the material territory of some key areas concerning treatment and prevention by re-thinking an information and flesh distinction.

In chapter 2, I asked: What are the implications of understanding science as performative for arresting HIV? In response, I noted that a performative account of science does not discount the presence of the virus or the work of ARVs. I argued that methodologies sufficiently reflexive to the performative work of science are necessary and may well enable urgently required new conceptual work. Nevertheless, as some may still ask, how will this achieve better drugs, diagnostics, conceptions of living with HIV? How will attention to our own performative work enable us to get beyond the constitutive work of power so insidiously materializing a world of givens that delimit the possibility of better drugs, diagnostics, and conceptions of living with HIV? Empirical answers to such questions are yet to follow. However, as I noted in the introduction, early cultural critiques give weight to their likelihood.

## THE OBJECT OF INQUIRY

A critique of objects and the question of how this is viable for science, a discipline more immediately perceived as directed toward the world of material objects than are others such as law, media, or social inquiry, has been central to this book. Because of this and Law and Urry's suggestion above that any intervention will be generative, I want to briefly consider then what might constitute an object for inquiry. I refer to Scott Lash and Celia Lury's recent proposal that an object may come to be recognized as such, that is, as separate, discrete or external: "at the moment at which [it] . . . acquired sufficient density of internal relations to emerge from its context; indeed, to be sufficiently robust so as to produce its own context, its own past, its own origin."[10] The object in this schema is not an enduring one and most certainly is open to change in its embodying of the performative process—intense as it may be—of its givenness. Indeed it is not unlike that of Butler and Barad's, although the Lash and Lury approach shifts emphasis to the object's motility. That is, Lash and Lury offer an account of an entity or object in movement, affected and affecting to include the researchers themselves, and this, I think, is an important note to finish on.

The following of an object on the basis of the relations responsible for its emergence or, in light of what I have said, its appearance at a given point in time and place, may be readily applied to the scientific object of HIV, originating with its identification as a retrovirus wreaking unceasing damage to a prior, yet continuing to be revised, conception of the immune system. It might also be applied to the person living with HIV and ARVs who—as Leila typifies—may be faced with considerations well in excess of the Trizivir slogan "I expect . . . my HIV treatment to be ongoing. Not always on my mind," discussed in chapter 3. Or, in fact, Trizivir itself may constitute an object. There is, in the terms of Lash and Lury, an abundance of objects comprising the epidemic, each bearing a sufficient density of internal relations to lead us to consider them as originary or self-identical. Most critically and ironically, from the perspective of this book, their contingent nature is highlighted by an abundance of scientific evidence. For example, I have shown here that ARVs do many things. They interfere with viral replication and in doing so prevent the onset of AIDS, but they also generate new forms of virus resistant to their work and, in numerous other ways, contribute to transformations of the "biological" and "social" of the field as captured, for example, in the statements of the self-identified gay men in chapter 4 or the clinical trials discussed in chapter 5.

Whether the objects of study are an HIV biotechnology or, further afield from what I have covered, another unwanted life-threatening condition or a prevention technology, each will take form through an interweaving of historical relations including those forged according to a presumption of independent observation. Whatever the virus is enacted or performed to be through state-of-the-art diagnostics, it is apparent from Leila's statement that these are part of her negotiation of the virus. They are integral to what are its effects. While these effects may be long-term depletion of the human immune system leading to AIDS, in her account it seems that there are other effects that matter. She wants confirmation of the presence of antibodies as evidence that she still has the virus. Antibodies provide a truth of status because they are a material or fleshed effect continuing to require investigation and justify treatment.

While much of this book has been in pursuit of "better biology," indicated by Haraway to be a strategy bound up in how the relationship of culture/ nature is understood, the key driver has been what I see as the need to re-think the ontological nature of HIV as it is already inscribed with the affective contributions of science and social science/humanities. It is on the basis of this recognition of the coextensive or intra-activity that new ways of conceptualizing HIV interventions are possible. Against the idea that HIV or, indeed, other infections or conditions are subject *to* intervention, there remains cause to reflect on how the infection or condition is already an effect of intervention. It is in the course of tracking this movement or traffic in information as flesh—that is, in our interventions—that something better may emerge.

# NOTES

## Chapter 1

The epigraph for this chapter is from R. Mitchell and P. Thurtle, *Data Made Flesh*, 1.

1 There are now numerous iterations of what a lay audience should understand as "HIV" and "AIDS." As one of the most authoritative, the Web site of the United States Government Centers for Disease Control and Prevention (CDC) states that "HIV (human immunodeficiency virus) is the virus that causes AIDS. This virus may be passed from one person to another when infected blood, semen, or vaginal secretions come in contact with an uninfected person's broken skin or mucous membranes. In addition, infected pregnant women can pass HIV to their baby during pregnancy or delivery, as well as through breast-feeding. People with HIV have what is called HIV infection. Some of these people will develop AIDS as a result of their HIV infection." AIDS is explained as follows: "AIDS stands for Acquired Immunodeficiency Syndrome. Acquired—means that the disease is not hereditary but develops after birth from contact with a disease causing agent (in this case, HIV). Immunodeficiency—means that the disease is characterized by a weakening of the immune system. Syndrome—refers to a group of symptoms that collectively indicate or characterize a disease. In the case of AIDS this can include the development of certain infections and/or cancers, as well as a decrease in the number of certain cells in a person's immune system. A diagnosis of AIDS is made by a physician using specific clinical or laboratory standards." See http://www.cdc.gov/hiv/resources/qa/qa1.htm.

2 F. J. Palella et al., "Declining Morbidity and Mortality among Patients with Advanced Human Immunodeficiency Virus Infection," *New England Journal of Medicine* 338 (1998): 853–60; Communicable Disease Surveillance Centre (CDSC), "Changes in the Incidence of AIDS and in AIDS Deaths: The Effects of Antiretroviral Treatment," *Communicable Disease Report* 7 (1997): 381.

3 For this reason it has been suggested that HIV/AIDS be renamed. R. E. Green and D. J. Ward, "Let's Call It HIV Infection, Not 'AIDS'" (Poster Presentation) 14th International AIDS Conference, AIDS 2002, Barcelona, Spain, 7–12 July 2002.

4 The phrase "full treatment access" is frequently used within the field to underscore that while there may be some form of medical treatment available, this

may not include ARVs or that ARVs may be available only to those who can afford them or have other means of access such as through their employment. According to the charity AVERTing HIV and AIDS, by the end of 2007, 7.1 million people were in immediate need of life-saving AIDS drugs in developing and transitional countries; of these, only 2.015 million (28 percent) were receiving the drugs. See http://www.avert.org/worldstats.htm.

5   For a comprehensive account of factors considered when treating with ARVs, see British HIV Association, "British HIV Association (BHIVA) Guidelines for the Treatment of HIV-1-Infected Adults with Antiretroviral Therapy," *HIV Medicine* 9 (2008): 563–608. Available online at http://www.bhiva.org/cms1191540.asp.

6   Post-Exposure Prophylaxis (PEP) involves the delivery of ARVs in a month course within 72 hours of possible exposure to HIV. See J. Richens, S. G. Edwards, and S. T. Sadiq, "Can the Promotion of Post-exposure Prophylaxis Following Sexual Exposure to HIV (PEPSE) Cause Harm?" *Sexually Transmitted Infections* 81 (2005): 190–91; J. Ghosn et al., on behalf of the British Co-operative Clinical Group of the Medical Society for the Study of Venereal Diseases, "Post-exposure Prophylaxis for Non-occupational Exposure to HIV: Current Clinical Practice and Opinions in the UK," *Sexually Transmitted Infections* 78, no. 2 (April 2002): 130–32.

7   I am deliberately using only the pronoun "he" because, to date, PEP has been debated in this way only in relation to the prevention needs of gay male communities.

8   Concerns over PEP are framed in a manner homologous to those raised in reference to other innovations in biotechnologies; consider, for example, questions about whether fertilized embryos should be used for research purposes; whether a deceased partner's sperm should be used in human reproduction; whether young girls will become sexually active before their natural time if they are immunized at puberty against cervical cancer; or whether there is cause for preventing the hybridization of a cow cell with human DNA in stem cell research. All of these queries are premised on the belief that biotechnologies are disruptive to accepted orderings of life and death, and that, consequently, these biotechnologies force us to address new social and ethical questions. But ignored in the framing of the technology as disruptive is its role in materializing the concern. For example, the very notion of an embryo, and its capacity to be materialized as an object of life for ethical consideration, is created in part by biotechnologies.

9   R. Mitchell and P. Thurtle, *Data Made Flesh*, 1. Innovations in biotechnologies reveal how the "seeming solid wall between bodies and information. . . bleeds; bodies and information continually graft themselves onto one another in a number of different cultural domains." The concept of a bleed gives emphasis to a dynamic taking place and notably involves a blurring of what otherwise

tends to be presumed as intractably apart. Although the distinction informs our practice and what we may understand as its effect, it is near impossible in conventional terms for one to be present without the other.

10  S. Franklin, C. Lury, and J. Stacey, *Global Nature, Global Culture* (Sage: London, 2000), 5.; Underpinning the critique I propose to take here is a complex history of debate on the nature of technology. The most recognizable tenet of this history is that the "matter" of the natural sciences—namely, "nature"—can no longer be sustained as invariably distinct from culture and as if prior to culture. The term "traffic," used here to convey a sense of productive or constitutive activity—even as it may lead to destruction and death—is adapted from Franklin, Lury, and Stacey's notion of "a traffic in nature" whereby a host of entities are de- and renaturalized as part of making the global. As they explain, traffic refers to "the constitutive effects of naturalized idioms as they are transferred across domains, revised, extended and made newly productive. . . ." In this constitutive movement between nature and culture, crossings with other seeming opposite pairs—such as nature and history and nature and technology—may also take place. Here I am interested in using the idea of traffic to de-naturalize a series of distinctions that tend to pass unchallenged within the HIV field, even as they are contradicted by knowledge produced and enacted within the field.

11  W. A. Haseltine and F. Wong-Staal, "The Molecular Biology of the AIDS Virus," *Scientific American* 259, no. 4 (1988): 34–42, quote is on p. 34.

12  C. Waldby, *The Visible Human Project: Informatic Bodies and Posthuman Medicine* (New York and London: Routledge, 2000), 25. This account need not be restricted to HIV, however. The body's molecular organization is increasingly available to being conceived as a cybernetic system.

13  See, for example, L. J. Picker and D. I. Watkins, "HIV Pathogenesis: The First Cut Is the Deepest," *Nature Immunology* 6, no. 5 (2005): 430–32. Although this is a generally accepted scientific understanding of HIV, this understanding does not preclude ongoing debate on the specific components that enable HIV in vivo.

14  See, for example, the discussion by R. Weiss, "Gulliver's Travels in HIVland," *Nature* 410 (2000): 963–67, in which HIV is noted as an ideal organism for genomics modeling because of the "data" it involves. Within the HIV field, although not in reference to ARVs, there are numerous accounts of HIV that presume it to be a biological entity engaged in information transmission.

15  UK Collaborative Group on Monitoring the Transmission of HIV Drug Resistance, "Analysis of Prevalence of HIV-1 Drug Resistance in Primary Infections in the United Kingdom," *British Medical Journal* 322 (2007): 1087–88.

16  See, for example, D. Haraway, "Situated Knowledges," *Simians, Cyborgs, and Women* (London: Free Association Books, 1991); and also H. Longino, "'Subjects, Power, and Knowledge: Description and Prescription in Feminist Philosophies

of Science," in *Feminism and Science*, ed. E. Fox Keller and H. Longino (Oxford: Oxford University Press, 1991).

17  D. Haraway discusses "the God's eye view" in her essay "Situated Knowledges," in *Simians, Cyborgs, and Women*, 189.

18  C. Patton, *Inventing AIDS* (New York and London: Routledge, 1990), 54.

19  Ibid., 55.

20  S. Watney, "The Spectacle of AIDS," in *The Lesbian and Gay Studies Reader*, ed. Henry Abelove, Michèle Aina Barale, and David M. Halperin (New York and London: Routledge, 1993), 203.

21  See Patton, *Inventing AIDS*, 27. Although gay men were not the only ones dying, they came to the attention of public health authorities as an anomaly. It was highly unusual to find young healthy men dying of rare cancers and pneumonias in contrast to an accepted level of disease presence among injecting drug users.

22  P. A. Treichler, "AIDS, Homophobia and Biomedical Discourse: An Epidemic of Signification," *October* 43 (Winter 1987): 31–70, quote is on p. 42.

23  J. Epstein, *Altered Conditions: Disease, Medicine and Storytelling* (New York and London: Routledge, 1995), 17.

24  Ibid., 171.

25  Ibid., 169.

26  In the United States, the Reagan administration refused to confirm that all individuals were at risk of HIV infection if they engaged in anal or vaginal intercourse without condoms or if they shared needles.

27  See Patton, "Inventing AIDS in Africa," in *Inventing AIDS*.

28  J. Butler, "Sexual Inversions," in *Discourses of Sexuality: From Aristotle to AIDS*, ed. Donna C. Stanton (Ann Arbor: University of Michigan Press, 1992), 345.

29  At the 16th International AIDS Conference in Toronto, Bill and Melinda Gates announced a commitment to supporting microbicide research. See http://www.cnn.com/2006/HEALTH/08/16/aids.transmission.cnn.

30  See S. Jintarkanon et al., "Unethical Clinical Trials in Thailand: A Community Response," *The Lancet* 3, no. 65 (2005): 1617–18. I am referring here to the undertaking of trials for a pre-exposure prophylaxis (PrEP) with people at risk of HIV infection from injecting drug use in a country where new needles have to be paid for. A US congressional ruling prohibits US aid being spent on the provision of these prophylactics within or outside a trial, even though this has been argued to contravene international ethics guidelines.

31  Institute of Science in Society, "Women Confront AIDS in Africa," Institute of Science in Society, http://www.i-sis.org.uk/Women_Confront_Aids_in_Africa.php.

32  T. Barnett and A. Whiteside, *AIDS in the Twenty-First Century: Disease and Globalization*, 2nd ed. (Basingstoke, UK: Palgrave Macmillan, 2006), 41.

33  J. Butler, *Bodies That Matter* (New York and London: Routledge, 1993), 35.

34  K. Race, "The Undetectable Crisis: Changing Technologies of Risk," *Sexualities* 4, no. 2 (2001): 167–89.

35  M. Fraser, "Standards, Populations, and Difference," ed. Brett Neilson, special issue, *Cultural Critique* (forthcoming).

36  B. Latour, *We Have Never Been Modern*, trans. C. Porter (Cambridge: Harvard University Press, 1993).

37  M. Callon, C. Méadel, and V. Rabeharisoa, "The Economy of Qualities," *Economy and Society* 31, no. 2, May (2002): 194–217.

38  See A. Barry, "Pharmaceutical Matters: The Invention of Informed Materials," in "Inventive Life: Approaches Towards a New Vitalism," ed. M. Fraser, S. Kember, and C. Lury, special issue, *Theory, Culture & Society* 22, no. 1 (2005): 51–69.

39  P. Rabinow, "Artificiality and Enlightenment: From Sociobiology to Biosociality," in *Essays on the Anthropology of Reason* (Princeton, NJ: Princeton University Press, 1996), 103.

40  Among the most illustrative materials underscoring the political nature of death was a Channel 4 program, "Dying for Drugs," produced by True Vision, directed by Brian Edwards, and shown on UK television in April 2003. Although it is outside the bounds of usual acceptability regarding broadcasting licenses, it showed how the denial of such a basic drug for thrush because of the exorbitant costs led to the starvation and death, on camera, of a small boy in Honduras. Fluconazole, when marketed under the trade name Diflucan by Pfizer, sells at US$29 a capsule, whereas the generic version at the time of the film was available in neighboring Guatemala at US$0.30 a capsule.

41  R. Diprose, *Corporeal Generosity: On Giving with Nietzsche, Merleau-Ponty, and Levinas* (Albany: State University of New York Press, 2002).

## Chapter 2

An earlier, and differently oriented, version of this chapter was published as "The Challenge of HIV for Feminist Theory," special issue, *Feminist Theory: Feminist Theory and/of Science* 5, no. 2 (2004): 205–22.

1   See A. Persson, "Incorporating Pharmakon: HIV, Medicine, and Body Shape Change," *Body & Society* 10, no. 4 (2004): 45–67; A. Persson, K. Race, and E. Wakeford, "Health in Context: Negotiating Medical Technology and Lived Experience," *Health: An Interdisciplinary Journal for the Social Study of Health, Illness and Medicine* 7, no. 4 (2003): 397–415. The range of known possible side effects is extensive. They can be the effect of an allergic reaction to the drug(s) or as a result of the toxicity of the drug itself.

2   British HIV Association (BHIVA), *HIV Medicine* 9 (2008): 563–608.

3   M. Rosengarten et al., "After the Euphoria: HIV Medical Technologies from the Perspective of Clinicians," *Sociology of Health and Illness* 26, no. 5 (2004): 575–96.

4    J. M. McCune, "The Dynamics of CD4 T-cell Depletion in HIV Disease," *Nature* 410 (2001): 974–79, quote is on p. 974.

5    J. Butler, *Bodies That Matter* (New York and London: Routledge, 1993), 1.

6    Ibid., 2.

7    Ibid.

8    Ibid., 9.

9    Ibid., 7.

10    Cheryl Chase, "Hermaphrodites with Attitude: Mapping the Emergence of Intersex Political Activism," *GLQ: A Journal of Lesbian and Gay Studies* 4, no. 2 (1998): 189–211.

11    This argument is elaborated in chapter 5 in reference to a binary conception of human host bodies.

12    Butler, *Bodies That Matter*, 35.

13    This distinction is taken from Vicki Kirby's critique of social constructionism. *Australian Feminist Studies* 14, no. 29 (1999): 19–29.

14    For a discussion on Butler in relation to social constructionism, see R. Herzig, "On Performance, Productivity, and Vocabularies of Motive in Recent Studies of Science," *Feminist Theory* 5, no. 2 (2004): 127–47.

15    Butler, *Bodies That Matter*, 5.

16    Kirby, "Human Nature," 20.

17    Kirby, "Human Nature," 27.

18    Ibid., 28. Emphasis in original.

19    Vicki Kirby, in M. Fraser, "What Is the Matter of Feminist Criticism," *Economy and Society* 31, no. 4 (2002): 606–25, quote is on p. 613.

20    I would like to acknowledge Helen Keane for bringing Kirby's contribution to my attention.

21    Fraser, "What Is the Matter of Feminist Criticism," 613.

22    "D. Haraway, *Simians, Cyborgs, and Women* (London: Free Association Books, 1991), 208. The term "material-semiotic" is from Donna Haraway who, in explicit reference to HIV, specifies bodies are not "ideological constructions" and states "a 'material-semiotic actor' is intended to highlight the object of knowledge as an active part of the apparatus of bodily production, without *ever* implying immediate presence of such objects or, what is the same thing, their final or unique determination of what can count as objective knowledge of a biomedical body at a particular historical juncture. . . . Their [bodies'] boundaries materialise in social interaction."

23    K. Barad, "Getting Real: Technoscientific Practices and the Materialization of Reality," *differences: A Journal of Feminist Cultural Studies* 10, no. 2 (1998): 87–128.

24    This might be considered a further development in the argument provided by Patton on science cited in chapter 1.

25    Barad, "Getting Real," 90, 91.

26    Butler, *Bodies That Matter*, 34, 35; see chapter 1, n. 34.

27 While this standpoint opens up a further realm of debate on what can be presumed "human" and especially given the argument by Kirby cited earlier on the problematic nature of assuming a distinction between nature and culture, it is clear that Barad wants more attention on an area that is lost when science presumes its work to be objective in a classical realist sense.

28 Barad, "Getting Real," 94.

29 Ibid., 93.

30 Ibid.

31 Butler, *Bodies That Matter*, 10.

32 See, for example, P. Flowers, "Gay Men and HIV/AIDS Risk Management," *Health* 5 (2001): 50–75; K. Race, "The Undetectable Crisis: Changing Technologies of Risk," *Sexualities* 4, no. 2 (2001): 167–89; S. Kippax and K. Race, "Sustaining Safe Practice: Twenty Years On," *Social Science & Medicine* 57 (2003): 1–12.

33 Patton, *Inventing AIDS*, 33, provides a helpful account of the tests used at the time and notes that, in practice, the test detects a chemical reaction to indicate that a certain biochemical process has occurred. It is on this basis antibodies are deduced.

34 The viral load test is understood to have been instrumental in the shift from ineffective monotherapy to effective combination therapy as it provided a different and, indeed, more effective knowledge of the virus. In contrast to the earlier hypothesized latent phase after initial infection, the viral load test was important in providing evidence that replication begins at the moment of infection. According to National AIDS Manual (NAM), "The use of viral load tests has also demonstrated that HIV is actively replicating inside the bodies of asymptomatic people from the moment of infection; at no time is the virus truly latent." See http://www.aidsmap.com/en/docs/6DF087FA-BF76-4957-8E6E-637D4840AE34.asp.

For one of the most significant articles challenging the latency theory, although some of the strategies for treating have since altered, see D. Ho, "Time to Hit HIV, Early and Hard," *New England Journal of Medicine* 333, no. 7 (1995): 450–51. However, for a more recent discussion of the more complex accounts of viral activity, see L. J. Picker and D. I. Watkins, "HIV Pathogenesis: The First Cut Is the Deepest," *Nature Immunology* 6, no. 5 (2005): 430–32.

35 I include the qualifier "credible" here to distinguish debate on how viral infection proceeds in vivo from the appropriation and dispute of the link between HIV and AIDS that has been put forward in spurious claims by J. Lauritsen, "First Things First: Some Thoughts on the 'AIDS Virus' and AZT," *New York Native* (1 June 1987): 14–16. The scientific discussion about a latent period is outlined by Steve Epstein and noted to have been based on a theory that there were three stages to infection: initial with a high viral load in the blood, then a latent period with low virus in the blood but gradual decline of T-cell count, fol-

lowed by the onset of opportunistic infections. S. Epstein, *Impure Science* (Berkeley: University of California Press, 1996), 283 and 316. It is also important to add that, at the time this book was going to press, new discussions were taking place amongst HIV scientists on the work of latent reservoirs within the body.

36  Epstein, *Impure Science,* 316.

37  Carefully calibrated measures have been established, mainly through clinical trials, to determine levels of both viral particles and CD4 in a blood sample to act as surrogate markers of disease progression. As noted in chapter 1, note 6, for a comprehensive account of factors considered when treating with ARVs, see British HIV Association, "British HIV Association (BHIVA) Guidelines for the Treatment of HIV-infected Adults with Antiretroviral Therapy," *HIV Medicine* 8 (2009): 563–608. Available online at http://www.bhiva.org/cms1222226.asp.

38  S. J. Little et al., "Antiretroviral-Drug Resistance among Patients Recently Infected with HIV," *New England Journal of Medicine* 34, no. 6 (8 August 2002): 385–94; S. Little, "Is Transmitted Drug Resistance in HIV on the Rise?" *British Medical Journal* 322 (2001): 1074–75.

39  For insight into how doctors view their patients and the basis for putting them on ARVs, see M. Rosengarten et al., "After the Euphoria," 575–96.

40  The phrase "chaotic" is sometimes used anecdotally as a euphemism for drug addiction.

41  M. A. Chesney et al., Patient Care Committee and Adherence Working Group of the Outcomes Committee of the Adult AIDS Clinical Trials Group (AACTG), "Self-reported Adherence to Antiretroviral Medications among Participants in HIV Clinical Trials: The AACTG Adherence Instruments," *AIDS Care* 12, no. 3 (2000): 255–66; K. Race and E. Wakeford, "Dosing on Time: Developing Adherent Practice with Highly Active Anti-retroviral Therapy," *Culture, Health & Sexuality* 2, no. 2 (2000): 213–28.

42  Race, "The Undetectable Crisis," 168.

43  Ibid., 177. In this essay Race makes the further and, indeed, more significant argument that the deployment of the viral load test produces a split whereby "health" (viral load test measure) is privileged over "well-being" (which may involve living with side effects). Pill count is therefore only one aspect of the ardors involved in fulfilling an ARV-instituted regime.

44  Race, "The Undetectable Crisis," 178.

45  M. A. Chesney et al., "Self-reported Adherence to Antiretroviral Medications," 255–66; G. Wagner, "Does Discontinuing the Use of Pill Boxes to Facilitate Electronic Monitoring Impede Adherence?" *International Journal of STD and AIDS* 14, no. 1 (2003): 64–65.

46  D. R. Bangsberg, A. R. Moss, and S. G. Deeks, "Paradoxes of Adherence and Drug Resistance to HIV Antiretroviral Therapy," *Journal of Antimicrobial Chemotherapy* 53 (2004): 696–99.

47  J. Schapiro, "Understanding Protease Inhibitor Potency: The Intersection of

Exposure, Efficacy, and Resistance," *The AIDS Reader* 11, no. 6 (2001): 311–15; K. Alcorn and R. Fieldhouse, eds., *AIDS Reference Manual* (London: National AIDS Manual Publications, December 2000), 157.

48 Schapiro, "Understanding Protease Inhibitor Potency," 312.

49 L. M. Frenkel and J. I. Mullins, "Should Patients with Drug-Resistant HIV-1 Continue to Receive Antiretroviral Therapy?" *New England Journal of Medicine* 344, no. 7 (2001): 520–22.

50 Schapiro, "Understanding Protease Inhibitor Potency," 312.

51 S. G. Deeks, T. Wrin, T. Liegler, R. Hoh, M. Hayden, J. D. Barbour, N. S. Hellmann, C. J. Petropoulos, J. M. McCune, M. K. Hellerstein, and R. M. Grant, "Virologic and Immunologic Consequences of Discontinuing Combination Antiretroviral-Drug Therapy in HIV-Infected Patients with Detectable Viremia," *New England Journal of Medicine* 7, no. 344 (2001): 472–80.

52 Following detection of increases in virus particles by the viral load test, other tests may be used to establish the nature of the mutated strain and sensitivity to other possible drugs.

53 M. A. Wainberg and G. Friedland, "Public Health Implications of Antiretroviral Therapy and HIV Drug Resistance," *Journal of American Medical Association* 279, no. 24 (1998): 1977–83.

54 At the time of writing, a group of Swiss-based researchers released the first-ever statement that they had evidence to show that individuals with an undetectable viral load and no STI cannot transmit HIV during sex. P. Vernazza et al., "Les personnes séropositives ne souffrant d'aucune autre MST et suivant un traitement antirétroviral efficace ne transmettent pas le VIH par voie sexuelle." *Bulletin des médecins suisses* 89, no. 5 (2008).

55 T. C. Quinn et al., "Viral Load and Heterosexual Transmission of Human Immunodeficiency Virus Type I," *New England Journal of Medicine* 342 (2000): 921–29.

## Chapter 3

This chapter is a revised version of the paper, "Consumer Activism in the Pharmacology of HIV," *Body & Society* 10, no. 1 (2004): 91–107.

The epigraph to this chapter is from P. A. Treichler, *How to Have Theory in an Epidemic: Cultural Chronicles of AIDS*, 329.

1 P. A. Treichler, *How to Have Theory in an Epidemic: Cultural Chronicles of AIDS* (Durham: Duke University Press, 1999), 329.

2 By linguistic I mean language in the more narrow conventional sense of speech and writing in contrast to an anthropological conception that might include other forms of communication such as food, kinship exchange, music, and dance.

3 Trizivir is made up of one class of antiretroviral drugs, nucleoside/nucleotide reverse transcriptase inhibitors (NRTIs).

4 M. Callon, C. Méadel, and V. Rabeharisoa, "The Economy of Qualities," *Economy and Society* 31, no. 2 (May 2002): 194–217, quote is on p. 194.

5 C. Patton, *Globalizing AIDS* (Minneapolis: University of Minnesota Press, 2002).

6 N. Rose and C. Novas, "Biological Citizenship" in *Global Assemblages: Technology, Politics and Ethics as Anthropological Problems*, ed. Aihwa Ong and Stephen Collier (Oxford: Blackwell, 2005), 439–63.

7 S. Epstein, *Impure Science* (Berkeley: University of California Press, 1996); C. Patton, "What 'Science' Knows about AIDS," in *Inventing AIDS* (New York and London: Routledge, 1990).

8 This has been particularly true of the Bill and Melinda Gates Foundation.

9 J. Butler, *Bodies That Matter* (New York and London: Routledge, 1993), 35.

10 Ibid., 34.

11 In contrast to the EU and Australia for instance, there is no restriction on prescription advertising to consumers in the United States and New Zealand.

12 R. Moynihan, I. Heath, and D. Henry, "Selling Sickness: The Pharmaceutical Industry and Disease Mongering," *British Medical Journal* 324 (2002): 886–91.

13 The expression "CD4 count" or "CD4 T-cell count" refers to a measure of the human immune cells that are understood to be most susceptible to destruction by the virus. Their decline allows for the advent of AIDS.

14 This discussion with the clinician was conducted while I was undertaking ethnographic research at a London clinic. Some of the material was later published in M. Rosengarten, J. Imrie, P. Flowers, M. D. Davis, and G. J. Hart, "After the Euphoria: HIV Medical Technologies from the Perspective of Clinicians," *Sociology of Health and Illness* 26, no. 5 (2004): 575–96.

15 Ibid.

16 R. Smith, "Medical Journals and Pharmaceutical Companies: Uneasy Bedfellows," *British Medical Journal* 326 (2003): 1202–5, quote is on p. 1202.

17 See, for example, L. Birke, A. Arluke, and M. Michael, *The Sacrifice: How Scientific Experiments Transform Animals and People* (West Lafayette, IN: Purdue University Press, 2006); for Sociology of Medicine, see J. Abraham and G. Lewis, "The Secrecy and Transparency of Medicines Licensing in the EU," *The Lancet* 352 no. 9 (8 August 1998): 480.

18 *British Medical Journal* 322 (20 January 2001): 126.

19 *Journal of the American Medical Association* 285, no. 1 (3 January 2001): 34.

20 For mention of this, see V. Nguyen, "Antiretroviral Globalism, Biopolitics, and Therapeutic Citizenship" in *Global Assemblages*, 140, 141.

21 *HIV Treatment Bulletin* 2, no. 1 (January/February 2001). Available online at http://www.i-base.info/pub/htb/vol2/htb2-1/htb2-1.html.

22 Ibid.

23  *+ve Magazine* 14, online issue, http://www.plusve.org/data/usercontentroot/ magazine/2001/issue%2014/default.asp.

24  *Positive Nation* 64 (2001): 35.

25  The financial incentive for speaking on behalf of a pharmaceutical product in this capacity is unknown. However, it is interesting to reflect on Ferner's summary of the UK Health Committee report, "The Influence of Big Pharma," editorial in *British Medical Journal* 33 (2006): 857–58. He notes that "key opinion leaders" may receive £5,000 for giving a lecture on behalf of a pharmaceutical company.

26  Although it is well acknowledged that many people with HIV are highly informed about antiretroviral combinations, this view should not be generalized to all those living with HIV in countries with full treatment access such as the UK or US.

27  For a discussion on the relationship between medical practitioners and pharmaceutical companies see R. Smith, "Medical Journals and Pharmaceutical Companies: Uneasy Bedfellows," *British Medical Journal* 326 (2003): 1202–5. See also D. Spurgeon, "Companies May Face Tighter Regulation over Promoting Drugs," *British Medical Journal* 329 (2004): 998. Spurgeon states that the industry spends "$12bn a year on gifts and payments to doctors; funds more than 70% of clinical trials, and shoulders more than half the costs of formal continuing education programmes in medicine." For a comprehensive account of how the relationship between "big pharma" and medicine turns on the role of the drug sales representative, see M. J. Oldani, "Thick Prescriptions: Toward an Interpretation of Pharmaceutical Sales Practices," *Medical Quarterly Anthropology* 18, no. 3 (September 2004): 325–56.

28  The UK-based treatment information organizations discussed here do not accept advertisements for ARVs.

29  BBC News, "Drug Simplifies Living with HIV," 16 January 2001, http://news. bbc.co.uk/hi/english/health/newsid_1119000/1119634.stm.

30  Ibid.

31  For a critique of the insistence on adherence, see K. Race, "The Undetectable Crisis: Changing Technologies of Risk," *Sexualities* 4, no. 2 (2001): 167–89.

32  W. Anderson and P. Weatherburn, *Taking Heart? The Impact of Combination Therapy on the Lives of People with HIV (Phase 2)* (London: Sigma Research, 1999).

33  Race, "The Undetectable Crisis," 181.

34  L. Adkins, "Objects of Innovation: Post-occupational Reflexivity and Re-traditionalisations of Gender," in *Transformations: Thinking Through Feminism*, ed. S. Ahmed, J. Kilby, C. Lury, M. McNeil, and B. Skeggs (New York and London: Routledge, 2000), 260.

35  See the discussion of Race's work in chapter 2 on the viral load test.

36  See Merck Web site, http://www.merck.com.

37  See Bristol-Myers Web site, http://www.bms.com/aboutbms/data.

38  See GlaxoSmithKline Web site, http://us.gsk.com/.

39  G. Deleuze and F. Guattari, *A Thousand Plateaus: Capitalism and Schizophrenia* (Minneapolis: University of Minnesota Press, 1988), 204.

40  The suggestion that drug regimes need to fit lifestyles is raised by C. Workman and R. Workman, whose work is discussed by K. Race and E. Wakeford in "Dosing on Time: Developing Adherent Practice with Highly Active Anti-retroviral Therapy," *Culture, Health & Sexuality* 2, no. 2 (2000): 213–28.

41  "Big pharma" sometimes offers the explanation that it is unable to provide ARVs at cost to developing countries because there is a lack of health care infrastructure to ensure the distribution.

## Chapter 4

1  S. G. Montaner et al., "The Case for Expanding Access to Highly Active Antiretroviral Therapy to Curb the Growth of the HIV Epidemic," *The Lancet* 368 (2006): 531–36.

2  According to H. W. Jaffe, R. O. Valdisseri, and K. M. De Cock, "The Reemerging HIV/AIDS Epidemic in Men Who Have Sex With Men," *Journal of the American Medical Association* 298 (2007): 2412, there was a reported 55 percent increase in new HIV cases of new infections among men who have sex with men (MSM) in thirteen western European countries between 1998 and 2005 and a 13 percent increase among MSM in the United States.

3  See, for example, S. Y. Chen, S. Gibson, and M. H. Katz, "Continuing Increases in Sexual Risk Behaviour and Sexually Transmitted Diseases among Men Who Have Sex with Men, San Francisco, 1999–2001," *American Journal of Public Health* 92 (2002): 1387–88; J. P. Dodds et al., "Increase in High Risk Sexual Behaviour among Homosexual Men, London 1996–8: Cross Sectional Questionnaire Study," *British Medical Journal* 320 (2000): 1510–11; N. H. T. M. Dukers et al., "Sexual Risk Behaviour Related to the Virological and Immunological Improvements during Highly Active Antiretroviral Therapy in HIV-1 Infection," *AIDS* 15 (2001): 369–78; P. Van de Ven et al., "Sexual Risk Behaviour Increases and Is Associated with HIV Treatment Optimism among HIV-negative and HIV-positive Gay Men in Sydney over the Four-year Period to February 2000," *AIDS* 14 (2000): 2952–53. Later it will become apparent that there are many different facets to this alteration in practice and thinking. It is important to note though that since the late 1990s and appearing to coincide with the introduction of ARVs in North America, western Europe, and Australia, behavioral surveillance has confirmed that the practice of anal intercourse without condoms, or more commonly referred to as unprotected anal intercourse or UAI, by gay men has become more frequent than earlier in the 1990s.

4  For a medical critique, see, for example, H. W. Jaffe, R. O. Valdisseri, and K. M. De Cock, "The Reemerging HIV/AIDS Epidemic in Men Who Have Sex with

Men," or for an overview and cultural analysis, see D. Halperin, *What Do Gay Men Want? An Essay on Sex, Risk, and Subjectivity* (Ann Arbor: University of Michigan Press, 2007).

5  See S. Kippax and K. Race, "Sustaining Safe Practice: Twenty Years On," *Social Science & Medicine* 57 (2003): 1–12.

6  M. Rosengarten, K. Race, and S. Kippax, "'Touch Wood, Everything Will Be OK': Gay Men's Understandings of Clinical Markers in Sexual Practise," *Monograph 7/2000* (Sydney: National Centre in HIV Social Research, 2000). Working closely with community organizations and gay-affiliated advisors to government, we reached the conclusion that knowledge of ARVs and associated tests provided a basis on which some gay men were able to devise more inventive and varied risk-minimization sexual strategies than those authorized by public health campaigns pre-ARVs. This conclusion drew on knowledge of the significance of the HIV antibody test (prior to the introduction of ARVs), according to which gay men were previously known to organize themselves in relation to conceptions of risk.

7  P. Van de Ven et al., "A Scale of Optimism-Scepticism in the Context of HIV Treatments," *AIDS Care* 12 (2000): 171–76; J. M. Stephenson et al., "Is Use of Antiretroviral Therapy among Homosexual Men Associated with Increased Risk of Transmission of HIV Infection?" *Sexually Transmitted Infections* 79 (2003): 7–10; J. Elford, G. Bolding, and L. Sherr, "High-risk Behavior Increases among London Gay Men between 1998 and 2001: What Is the Role of HIV Optimism?" *AIDS* 16 (2002): 1537–44.

8  Kippax and Race, "Sustaining Safe Practice," 4. This observation can be made of gay men since the beginning of the epidemic.

9  See, for example, N. Sheon and G. M. Crosby, "Ambivalent Tales of HIV Disclosure in San Francisco," *Social Science & Medicine* 58 (2004): 2105–18.

10  J. Richens, S. G. Edwards, and S. T. Sadiq, "Can the Promotion of Post-exposure Prophylaxis Following Sexual Exposure to HIV (PEPSE) Cause Harm?" *Sexually Transmitted Infections* 81 (2005): 190–91. For an alternate argument, see C. R. Waldo, R. D. Stall, and T. J. Coates, "Is Offering Post-Exposure Prevention for Sexual Exposures to HIV Related to Sexual Risk Behaviour in Gay Men? *AIDS* 14 (2000): 1035–39.

11  See, for example, R. O. Valdiserri, "Mapping the Roots of HIV/AIDS Complacency: Implications for Program and Policy Development," *AIDS Education and Prevention* 16, no. 5 (2004): 426–39; B. Adam, "Infection Behaviour: Imputing Subjectivity to HIV Transmission," *Social Theory & Health* 4 (2006): 168–79.

12  K. Race, "Revaluation of Risk among Gay Men," *AIDS Education and Prevention* 4 (2003): 369–81, quote is on p. 377.

13  A. Barry, "Pharmaceutical Matters: The Invention of Informed Materials," in "Inventive Life: Approaches Towards a New Vitalism," ed. M. Fraser, S. Kember, and C. Lury, special issue, *Theory, Culture & Society* 22, no. 1 (2005): 51–69, quote is on p. 52.

14  Ibid., 55.

15  A. N. Whitehead, cited in Barry, "Pharmaceutical Matters," 56.

16  A. N. Whitehead, *Science and the Modern World* (London: Free Association, 1985), 23.

17  Barry, "Pharmaceutical Matters," 58.

18  Ibid., 59.

19  Although of late, the current Bush administration has significantly undermined this with a funding policy that carries the caveat that funding for HIV prevention must promote abstinence in place of condoms and not sharing needles.

20  Kippax and Race, "Sustaining Safe Practice," 9.

21  For a detailed account of the United States government's response to the epidemic, see P. Treichler, *How to Have Theory in an Epidemic: Cultural Chronicles of AIDS* (Durham, NC: Duke University Press, 1999), 57.

22  See C. Patton, "Inventing 'African AIDS.'" Chapter 4 in *Inventing AIDS* (New York and London: Routledge, 1990); see P. Triechler, "Beyond Cosmo: AIDS, Identity, and Inscriptions of Gender." Chapter 8 in *How to Have Theory in an Epidemic,* on the effects of homophobia on the treatment of women and their exclusion from effective prevention messages.

23  Judith Butler provides a detailed discussion of the homophobic treatment of gays but also the broader designating of people with AIDS as abject in *Gender Trouble: Feminism and the Subversion of Identity* (New York and London: Routledge, 1990), 132, 133.

24  Butler, *Bodies That Matter: On the Discursive Limits of Sex* (New York and London: Routledge, 1993), 8.

25  See http://www.markichester.com for the full series by Chester.

26  J. Grover, "OI: Opportunistic Identification, Open Identification in PWA Portraiture," in *Don't Leave Me This Way: Art in the Age of AIDS*, compiled by Ted Gott (Melbourne: National Gallery of Australia; London and New York: Thames and Hudson, 1994), 226, 227.

27  See D. Crimp, "Portraits of People with AIDS," in *Cultural Studies*, ed. L. Grossberg, C. Nelson, and P. Treichler (New York and London: Routledge, 1992). ACT UP is an activist organization currently most established and operative in France and the United States. It commenced in the early 1980s and produced public art including slogans to challenge homophobia and the neglect of HIV/AIDS.

28  J. Grover, "OI," 227.

29  This statement by David McDiarmid is from a Web site celebrating a retrospective of his work. He was commenting on his poster series commissioned by the AIDS Action Council of New South Wales in 1992. See http://www.aidsaction.org.au/content/events/reflections/there_isnt_room_for_ambiguity.php.

30  Kippax and Race, "Sustaining Safe Practice," 2. This statement was also included on the above Web site for the David McDiarmid retrospective. It is well

supported, however. Indeed, Kippax and Race note that not only in Australia but in most northern European countries, and among some populations in the United States and Canada, HIV rates declined. Kippax and Race add a caveat to this by noting also that the earliest effective prevention efforts were produced by gay men and injecting drug users.

31 Besides identifying as gay, each person was asked to self-nominate for the research according to their known or perceived serostatus (for some who identified as HIV-negative, this was based on an unlikely to have altered test result, for others their HIV-negative status was not so certain).

32 Barry, "Pharmaceutical Matters," 56; A. N. Whitehead, *Science and the Modern World*, 136.

33 D. Murphy, "Risk Reduction Strategies for Anal Sex with Casual Partners," *AFAO/NAPWA Education Discussion Paper* 2, no. 4 (2000/2001). According to the *Guidelines for the Management and Post Exposure Prophylaxis of Individuals Who Sustain Nonoccupational Exposure to HIV, ANCAHRD/CTARC Bulletin*, February 2001, the risk of transmission as a result of receptive anal sex is 1:125 to 1:31 or approximately 3 percent; for insertive anal sex, the risk is 1:3333 to 1:1111 or approximately 0.1 percent. However, given the seemingly increasing trend toward differentiating risk according to receptive or insertive positions, it is important to stress here that epidemiological risk is a statistical measure. Indeed, there is no certainty that an HIV-negative individual will be safe from infection by being the insertive partner.

34 P. Van de Ven et al., "In a Minority of Gay Men, Sexual Risk Practice Indicates Strategic Positioning for Perceived Risk Reduction Rather Than Unbridled Sex," *AIDS Care* 14 (2002): 471–80.

35 See D. T. Ridge, "'It Was an Incredible Thrill': The Social Meanings and Dynamics of Younger Gay Men's Experiences of Barebacking in Melbourne," *Sexualities* 7, no. 3 (2004): 259–79. Although the term is not used directly, this type of fatigue is also discussed in the article by N. Sheon and G. M. Crosby, "Ambivalent Tales of HIV Disclosure in San Francisco," 2110.

36 In Australia, the term "safe" sex has been used throughout the epidemic, whereas the term "safer" has been and continues to be used in the UK .

37 Kippax and Race, "Sustaining Safe Practice," 7; Sheon and Crosby, "Ambivalent Tales of HIV Disclosure in San Francisco," 2105.

38 A. Mol, *The Body Multiple: Ontology in Medical Practice* (Durham, NC: Duke University Press, 2003).

39 See L. Mao et al., "'Serosorting' in Casual Anal Sex of HIV-negative Gay Men Is Noteworthy and Is Increasing in Sydney, Australia," *AIDS* 20, no. 8 (12 May 2006): 1204–6. The practice of "serosorting"—whereby individuals seek out another or others of the same HIV antibody status—allows for the forgoing of condoms in an intended non-risky manner. Not surprisingly it is contentious. Ensuring a partner of the same status—especially within casual relations but,

not exclusively, as "stable" heterosexual relations indicate—is not entirely reliable. However, an alternative strategy whereby people of HIV-negative status use antibody testing and the ideal of trust to serosort has been recognized since before ARVs.

40  See Barry, "Pharmaceutical Matters," 57. Being an "informed embodied subject" is to embody the context in which one is being informed or, as Andrew Barry says, in reference to atoms and molecules, the informational context "enters into the constitution of an entity."

41  B. Adam, "Constructing the Neoliberal Sexual Actor," *Culture, Health & Sexuality* 7, no. 4 (2005): 333–46. See for a valuable discussion of how the populist term "barebacking" to refer to UAI might be understood in ways similar to what I am suggesting here, except without inclusion of the significance of biomedically altered virus and body.

42  Unpublished interview material with people who had undergone a course of HIV post-exposure prophylaxis, on what they believed resulted in their taking risk, was incorporated to help us gain further insight into gay men's thinking on medical technologies and risk. The suggestion to incorporate this material was provided by Susan Kippax, the principal investigator of our study.

43  See note 5.

44  Law and Urry, "Enacting the Social," 398.

45  P. Flowers, "Gay Men and HIV/AIDS Risk Management," *Health* 5, no. 1 (2001): 50–75. This reading of the field might be extended much more widely than Australia. In this article, Flowers discusses Peter Keogh's (1996) study of 233 posters, postcards, and leaflets targeting gay men's sexual health from around Europe, Australia, and the United States that found that HIV prevention materials have been almost entirely focused upon the perspectives of the uninfected; those men who were HIV-negative/or untested.

46  An argument for how the notion of responsibility pervades the gay sexual culture is provided by Barry Adam, "Constructing the Neoliberal Sexual Actor," 344. Adam argues that "barebacking," the term commonly used to refer to UAI, involves a neoliberal subject who thinks in terms of consent, free market choice, and contractual interaction with versions of responsibilized activity based on these.

47  Kippax and Race, "Sustaining Safe Practice," 8.

48  M. Michael, *Technoscience and Everyday Life: The Complex Simplicities of the Mundane* (Berkshire, England: Open University Press, 2006), 115.

49  Adam, "Constructing the Neoliberal Sexual Actor," 339.

50  Will said that his partner did not seroconvert after this experience. Possibly, given Will's role as the insertive partner, the risk of seroconversion was averted due to Will's low viral load and his "guess" that he was probably not infectious.

## Chapter 5

The epigraphs are drawn from Judith Butler, *Bodies That Matter: On the Discursive Limits of Sex* (New York and London: Routledge, 1993), 8; and Donna J. Haraway, *Modest_Witness@Second_Millennium: FemaleMan@_MeetsOncoMouse™* (New York and London: Routledge, 1997), 213.

1   See A. Barry, "Pharmaceutical Matters: The Invention of Informed Materials," in "Inventive Life: Approaches Towards a New Vitalism," ed. M. Fraser, S. Kember, and C. Lury, special issue, *Theory, Culture & Society* 22, no. 1 (2005): 51–69; K. Barad, "Getting Real: Technoscientific Practices and the Materialization of Reality," *differences: A Journal of Feminist Cultural Studies* 10, no. 2 (1998): 87–128. According to my argument in chapters 3 and 4, the very notion of "object" must acquire new meaning.

2   S. Epstein, "Bodily Differences and Collective Identities: The Politics of Gender and Race in Biomedical Research in the United States," *Body & Society* 10, no. 2–3 (2004): 183–203, see p. 184.

3   Epstein, "Bodily Differences and Collective Identities," 184, notes that in the US, women "whether pregnant or not, or had any intention of becoming so, out of concern that an experimental drug might bring harm to a foetus" had been excluded from medical trials since 1977. With regard to other groups, their absence has a more complex history than what might appear as neglect. Members of presumed racial categories and, most specifically African Americans, were often highly wary of medical studies as the latter had used people racially identified for experimental purposes, for example with the Tuskegee Syphilis Study during which African Americans were not told they were infected with syphilis so that their disease progression could be studied. See G. Corbie-Smith, "The Continuing Legacy of the Tuskegee Syphilis Study: Considerations for Clinical Investigation," *American Journal of the Medical Sciences* 317 (1999): 5–8.

4   Epstein, "Bodily Differences and Collective Identities," 192.

5   This extract is taken from the National Health Institutes Web site, http://grants.nih.gov/grants/funding/phs398/instructions2/p2_nih_policy_report_race_ethnicity.htm, cited March 2006.

6   S. de Beauvoir, *The Second Sex,* trans. H. M. Parshley (London: Picador, 1988).

7   CDC, http://www.cdc.gov/od/foia/policies/inclusio.htm, cited 1 April 2006.

8   See Epstein, "Bodily Differences and Collective Identities," 183. The US National Institute of Health (NIH) is noted to be the world's largest funder of medical research.

9   See, for example, C. Patton, *Inventing AIDS* (New York and London: Routledge, 1990), 78–97; Patton, *Globalizing AIDS* (Minneapolis: University of Minnesota Press, 2002); D. Fassin, *When Bodies Remember: Experiences and Politics of AIDS in South Africa* (Berkeley: University of California Press, 2007); Treichler, "AIDS, Africa, and Cultural Theory," in *How to Have Theory in an Epidemic: Cultural*

*Chronicles of AIDS* (Durham, NC: Duke University Press, 1999), 205–34.

10  J. Butler, *Bodies That Matter*, 8.

11  In 2003, 58 percent of the 26.6 million people living with HIV/AIDS in sub-Saharan Africa were women. In Africa, young women (15–24) are 2.5 times more likely to have HIV than young men. See *Fact Sheet 4: Gender Equality in AIDS Protection* (Global Microbicide Campaign), 2005. In the United Kingdom, the pattern of infection has shifted from increases among gay men to heterosexual men and women. See AVERT, http://www.avert.org/uksummary.htm, cited June 2005.

12  This is a view expressed by Stephen Lewis, UN Special Envoy for HIV/AIDS in Africa, in a speech he delivered at the University of Pennsylvania's Summit on Global Issues in Women's Health, Philadelphia, 26 April 2005.

13  Bill Gates, of the Bill and Melinda Gates Foundation, announced at the International AIDS Conference held in Toronto in 2006 that his foundation would be increasing its funding of microbicide research as new prevention technologies are imperative and the development of vaccines is anticipated to take many more years. Gates stated, "Microbicides and oral prevention drugs could be the next big breakthrough in the fight against AIDS." See http://www.seedmagazine.com/news/2006/08/at_aids_conference_vaccines_ta.php.

14  T. M. Exner, S. Hoffman, S. Dworkin, and A. A. Ehrhardt. "Beyond the Male Condom: The Evolution of Gender-Specific HIV Interventions for Women." *Annual Review of Sex Research* 14 (2003): 114–36.

15  For statistics on this in the context of an innovative discussion of the work of epidemiology in producing the object it claims to report on, see S. L. Dworkin, "Who Is Epidemiologically Fathomable in the HIV/AIDS Epidemic? Gender, Sexuality, and the Intersectionality in Public Health," *Culture, Health & Sexuality* 7 (Nov.–Dec. 2005): 615–23.

16  P. An et al., "Influence of CCR5 Promoter Haplotypes on AIDS Progression in African-Americans," *AIDS* 14 (2000): 2117–22, quote is on p. 2121.

17  This quote is from C. Winkler, Ping An, and S. J. O'Brien, "Patterns of Ethnic Diversity among the Genes That Influence AIDS," *Human Molecular Genetics* 13, Review Issue 1 (2004): R9–R19, quote is on p. R16. Alleles are forms of genes whose location on a chromosome informs body phenomena, for example, at a locus for eye color the allele might result in blue or brown eyes.

18  For a discussion on Heidegger and Latour's conception of this, see Adrian Mackenzie, *Transductions: Bodies and Machines at Speed* (London and New York: Continuum, 2002), 7.

19  For such evidence, see, for example, P. Bieniasz, *New Insights into Retrovirus-host-cell Interactions*, 15th Conference on Retroviruses and Opportunistic Infections, Boston, abstract 114, 2008; J. Guatelli, D. Goff, and N. Van Damme, *Modulation of Viral Assembly and Virion Release by Vpu*, 15th Conference on Retroviruses and Opportunistic Infections, Boston, abstract 104a, 2008; E. Check, "Hunt for AIDS Vaccine Tackles Genomes," *Nature* 441 (2006): 1034–35.

20 By introducing the analytic concept of relationality, I will be bringing Butler's theory of performativity into a dialogue of sorts with the more biotechnologically oriented critique of Barad and those developed through Whitehead's work on relationality and process.

21 V. Satya Suresh Attili et al., "Validity of Existing CD4+ Classification in North Indians, in Predicting Immune Status," *Journal of Infection* 51 (2002): 41–46.

22 Attili et al., "Validity of Existing CD4+ Classification in North Indians, in Predicting Immune Status," 42.

23 N. Risch, E. Burchard, E. Ziv, and H. Tang, "Categorization of Humans in Biomedical Research: Genes, Race and Disease," *Genome Biology* 3, no. 7 (2002): comment 2007.1–2007.12 cited in M. Fraser, "Standards, Populations, and Difference,," ed. Brett Neilson, special issue, *Cultural Critique* (forthcoming).

24 A. N. Whitehead, *Process and Reality*, ed. David Ray Griffin and Donald W. Sherburne (New York and London: Free Press, 1978), 18.

25 Fraser, citing Delanda, in "Standards, Populations, and Difference." 26 Fraser, "Standards, Populations, and Difference," 2.

27 Butler, *Bodies That Matter*, 34.

28 For a discussion of Whitehead and values, see M. Fraser, "The Ethics of Reality and Virtual Reality: Latour, Facts and Values," *History of the Human Sciences* 19 (2006): 45–72, see p. 58.

29 Butler, *Bodies That Matter*, 1–2.

30 E. B. Burchard et al., "The Importance of Race and Ethnic Background in Biomedical Research and Clinical Practice," *New England Journal of Medicine* 348, no. 12 (2003): 1170–76.

31 See T. R. Sterling et al., "Initial Plasma HIV-1 RNA Levels and Progression to AIDS in Women and Men," *New England Journal of Medicine* 344, no. 10 (2001): 720–25. Assessment of viral progression is made by considering the measures of viral load and CD4 T-cells. Of late, a sufficient number of CD4 T-cells is considered more important than the level of viral load or measure of viral particles. That is, if the human immune system appears to have sufficient cells for fighting disease, then high levels of virus may not be a concern.

32 S. L. Dworkin, "Who Is Epidemiologically Fathomable in the HIV/AIDS Epidemic? Gender, Sexuality, and the Intersectionality in Public Health," 616.

33 R. W. Coombs et al., "A Comparison of HIV-1 Level in Blood and Non-Blood Compartments between Men and Women: Baseline Analysis of ACTG Protocol A5077," 44th Interscience Conference on Antimicrobial Agents and Chemotherapy, Washington, abstract H-198, 2004.

34 CASCADE Collaboration, "Differences in CD4 Cell Counts at Seroconversion and Decline among 5739 HIV-1-Infected Individuals with Well-Estimated Dates of Seroconversion," *Journal of Acquired Immune Deficiency Syndrome* 34, no. 1 (2003): 76–83, see 77, 78, 79.

35 Ibid., 80, 81.

36  R. Gray et al., "Increased Risk of Incident HIV during Pregnancy in Rakai, Uganda: A Prospective Study," *The Lancet* 366, no. 9492 (2005): 1182–88.

37  In this statement Epstein references the work of B. Hanson, "Bodily Differences and Collective Identities: The Politics of Gender and Race in Biomedical Research in the United States," in *Social Assumptions, Medical Categories* (Greenwich, CT: JAI Press, 1997), 195.

38  C. Chase, "Hermaphrodites with Attitude: Mapping the Emergence of Intersex Political Activism," *GLQ: A Journal of Lesbian and Gay Studies* 4, no. 2 (1998): 189–211.

39  In the case of hermaphrodites, it is now believed in some areas of medical science that the fusing of twin embryos into one surviving child may result in two sets of sex organs (sometimes the "same" and sometimes of the "opposite" sex).

40  M. Hird, "Chimerism, Mosaicism and the Cultural Construction of Kinship," *Sexualities* 7, no. 2 (2004): 217–32, states that chimerism is more likely associated with xenotransplantation (non-human organs into human) or transplantation although it can be a hereditary phenomena as is mosaicism that refers to patches of tissue that differ genetically. Hird cites figures that suggest as many as 4 percent of twins and 14 percent of triplet individuals are chimeras. She adds that there is a probable higher but unknown incidence of the phenomena within the general population.

41  B. Latour, "How to Talk About the Body? The Normative Dimension of Science Studies," *Body & Society* 10, no. 2–3 (2004): 205–29.

42  Ibid., 206.

43  Scott, cited in Reardon, "Decoding Race and Human Difference in a Genomic Age," 41.

## Conclusion

1  In the clinical management of HIV, the most significant surrogate of viral progression is not viral load but CD4 T-cell counts. The latter are the critical part of the human immune system depleted by HIV and, in their absence, AIDS is likely to occur.

2  C. Patton, *Globalizing AIDS* (Minneapolis: University of Minnesota Press, 2002).

3  E. Cameron, with contributions by Nathan Geffen, *Witness to AIDS* (Capetown: Tafelberg, 2005), 43.

4  K. Race, "The Undetectable Crisis: Changing Technologies of Risk," *Sexualities* 4, no. 2 (2001): 167–89.

5  C. Novas and N. Rose, "Genetic Risk and the Birth of the Somatic Individual," special issue, *Economy and Society* 29, no. 4 (2000): 484–513, see p. 488.

6  In raising these aspects of living with HIV I do not want to imply that negotiating safe sex or preventing mother to child transmission are necessarily difficult,

rather that there are further areas where a specific set of considerations and consequences emerge.

7   For a discussion of the contributions of Heidgegger and Latour, among others, on the question of technology, see A. Mackenzie, *Transductions: Bodies and Machines at Speed* (London and New York: Continuum, 2002), 7.

8   J. Law and J. Urry, "Enacting the Social," *Economy and Society* 33, no. 3 (August 2004): 390–410.

9   C. Lury, "From Diversity to Heterogeneity: A Feminist Analysis of the Making of Kinds," *Economy and Society* 31, no. 4 (2002): 588–605; see especially p. 590 for the reference to Donna Haraway's argument on what Lury describes as the enterprising of what has been nature in a cultural commodity, as in the case of Dupont's breeding of "oncomouse" for cancer drug testing or Monsanto's breeding of a potato that farmers cannot reproduce. Lury's own work concerns how the fashion brand Benneton has commodified race as a style of choice.

10  S. Lash and C. Lury, *Global Culture Industries: The Mediation of Things* (Cambridge and Malden: Polity Press, 2007), 23.

# Bibliography

Abraham, J., and G. Lewis. "The Secrecy and Transparency of Medicines Licensing in the EU." *The Lancet* 352, no. 9126 (8 August 1998): 480–82.

Adam, B. "Constructing the Neoliberal Sexual Actor." *Culture, Health & Sexuality* 7, no. 4 (2005): 333–46.

———. "Infection Behaviour: Imputing Subjectivity to HIV transmission." *Social Theory & Health* 4 (2006): 168–79.

Adkins, L. "Objects of Innovation: Post-occupational Reflexivity and Re-traditionalisations of Gender." In *Transformations: Thinking Through Feminism*, edited by S. Ahmed, J. Kilby, C. Lury, M. McNeil, and B. Skeggs. New York and London: Routledge, 2000.

AIDS Action Council of New South Wales. "there isn't room for ambiguity," http://www.aidsaction.org.au/content/events/reflections/there_isnt_room_for_ambiguity.php, 1992.

AIDS Vaccine Advocacy Coalition (AVAC). "Will a Pill a Day Prevent HIV? Anticipating the Results of 'PREP' Trials." New York: AVAC AIDS Vaccine Advocacy Coalition, 2005.

Alcorn, K., and R. Fieldhouse. *AIDS Reference Manual*. London: NAM Publications, 2000.

An, P., M. P. Martin, G. W. Nelson, M. Carrington, M. W. Smith, K. Gong, D. Vlahov, S. J. O'Brien, and C. A. Winkler. "Influence of CCR5 Promoter Haplotypes on AIDS Progression in African-Americans." *AIDS* 14 (2000): 2117–22.

Anderson, W., and P. Weatherburn. *Taking Heart? The Impact of Combination Therapy on the Lives of People with HIV (Phase 2)*. London: Sigma Research, 1999.

Attili, V. S. S., S. Sundar, V. P. Singh, and M. Rai. "Validity of Existing CD4+ Classification in North Indians, in Predicting Immune Status." *Journal of Infection* 51 (2002): 41–46.

AVERT an international AIDS charity: http://www.avert.org/aids-africa-questions-2.htm.

Bangsberg, D. R., A. R. Moss, and S. G. Deeks. "Paradoxes of Adherence and Drug Resistance to HIV Antiretroviral Therapy." *Journal of Antimicrobial Chemotherapy* 53 (2004): 696–99.

Barad, K. "Getting Real: Technoscientific Practices and the Materialization of Reality." *differences: A Journal of Feminist Cultural Studies* 10, no. 2 (1998): 87–128.

Barnett, T., and A. Whiteside. *AIDS in the Twenty-First Century: Disease and Globalization,* 2nd ed. Basingstoke, UK: Palgrave Macmillan, 2006.

Barry, A. "Pharmaceutical Matters: The Invention of Informed Materials." In "Inventive Life: Approaches Towards a New Vitalism," special issue edited by M. Fraser, S. Kember, and C. Lury, *Theory, Culture & Society* 22, no. 1 (2005): 51–69.

Bieniasz, P. *New Insights into Retrovirus-host-cell Interactions.* 15th Conference on Retroviruses and Opportunistic Infections, Boston, abstract 114, 2008.

Birke, L., A. Arluke, and M. Michael. *The Sacrifice: How Scientific Experiments Transform Animals and People.* West Lafayette, IN: Purdue University Press, 2006.

BBC News. "Drug Simplifies Living with HIV. "16 January 2001, http://news.bbc.co.uk/hi/english/health/newsid_1119000/1119634.stm.

Bristol-Myers Web site. http://www.bms.com/aboutbms/data.

British HIV Association. "British HIV Association (BHIVA) Guidelines for the Treatment of HIV-1-Infected Adults with Antiretroviral Therapy." *HIV Medicine* 9 (2008): 563–608.

Burchard, E. B., E. Ziv, N. Coyle, S. L. Gomez, et al. "The Importance of Race and Ethnic Background in Biomedical Research and Clinical Practice." *New England Journal of Medicine* 348, no. 12 (2003): 1170–76.

Butler, J. *Bodies That Matter: On the Discursive Limits of Sex.* New York and London: Routledge, 1993.

———. *Gender Trouble: Feminism and the Subversion of Identity.* New York and London: Routledge, 1990.

———. *Psychic Power of Life: Theories in Subjection.* Stanford, CA: Stanford University Press, 1997.

———. "Sexual Inversions." In *Discourses of Sexuality: From Aristotle to AIDS*, edited by D. Stanton. Ann Arbor: University of Michigan Press, 1992.

Callon, M., C. Mèadel, and V. Rabeharisoa. "The Economy of Qualities." *Economy and Society* 31, no. 2 (2002): 194–217.

Cameron, E., with contributions by N. Geffen. *Witness to AIDS.* Capetown: Tafelberg, 2005.

CASCADE Collaboration. "Differences in CD4 Cell Counts at Seroconversion and Decline Among 5739 HIV-1-Infected Individuals with Well-Estimated Dates of Seroconversion." *Journal of Acquired Immune Deficiency Syndrome* 34, no. 1 (2003): 76–83.

CDC (Communicable Disease Surveillance Centre). "Changes in the Incidence of AIDS and in AIDS Deaths: The Effects of Antiretroviral Treatment." *CDR* 7 (1997): 381.

CDC (Centers for Disease Control and Prevention). "What Is HIV?" http://www.cdc.gov/hiv/resources/qa/qa1.htm.

Chase, C. "Hermaphrodites with Attitude: Mapping the Emergence of Intersex Political Activism." *GLQ: A Journal of Lesbian and Gay Studies* 4, no. 2 (1998): 189–211.

Check, E. "Hunt for AIDS Vaccine Tackles Genomes." *Nature* 441 (2006): 1034–35.

Chen, S. Y., S. Gibson, and M. H. Katz. "Continuing Increases in Sexual Risk Behaviour and Sexually Transmitted Diseases among Men Who Have Sex with Men, San Francisco, 1999–2001." *American Journal of Public Health* 92 (2002): 1387–88.

Chesney, M. A., J. R. Ickovics, D. B. Chambers, A. L. Gifford, J. Neidig, B. Zwickl, and A. W. Wu. Patient Care Committee and Adherence Working Group of the Outcomes Committee of the Adult AIDS Clinical Trials Group (AACTG). "Self-reported Adherence to Antiretroviral Medications among Participants in HIV Clinical Trials: The AACTG Adherence Instruments." *AIDS Care* 12, no. 3 (2000): 255–66.

Coombs, R.W., et al. "A Comparison of HIV-1 Level in Blood and Non-blood Compartments between Men and Women: Baseline Analysis of ACTG Protocol A5077." 44th Interscience Conference on Antimicrobial Agents and Chemotherapy, Washington, abstract H-198, 2004.

Corbie-Smith, G. "The Continuing Legacy of the Tuskegee Syphilis Study: Considerations for Clinical Investigation." *American Journal of the Medical Sciences* 317 (1999): 5–8.

Court, M. "GSK AIDS Drug Approved." *The Times*, 5 January 2001, cited at www.thetimes.co.uk.

Crimp, D. "Portraits of People with AIDS." In *Cultural Studies*, edited by L. Grossberg, C. Nelson, and P. Treichler. New York and London: Routledge, 1992.

de Beauvoir, S. *The Second Sex.* Trans. H. M. Parshley. London: Picador, 1988.

Deeks, S. G., T. Wrin, T. Liegler, R. Hoh, M. Hayden, J. D. Barbour, N. S. Hellmann, C. J. Petropoulos, J. M. McCune, M. K. Hellerstein, and R. M. Grant. "Virologic and Immunologic Consequences of Discontinuing Combination Antiretroviral-Drug Therapy in HIV-Infected Patients with Detectable Viremia." *New England Journal of Medicine* 7, no. 344 (2001): 472–80.

Deleuze, G., and F. Guattari. *A Thousand Plateaus: Capitalism and Schizophrenia.* Trans. and with a foreword by Brian Massumi. Minneapolis: University of Minnesota Press, 1988.

Diprose, R. *Corporeal Generosity: On Giving with Nietzsche, Merleau-Ponty, and Levinas.* Albany: State University of New York Press, 2002.

Dodds J. P., A. Nardone, D. E. Mercey, and A. M. Johnson. "Increase in High Risk Sexual Behaviour among Homosexual Men, London 1996–8: Cross Sectional Questionnaire Study." *British Medical Journal* 320 (2000): 1510–11.

Dukers, N. H. T. M, J. Goudsmit, J. B. de Wit, M. Prins, et al. "Sexual Risk Behaviour Related to the Virological and Immunological Improvements during Highly Active Antiretroviral Therapy in HIV-1 Infection." *AIDS* 15 (2001): 369–78.

Dworkin, S. L. "Who is Epidemiologically Fathomable in the HIV/AIDS Epidemic? Gender, Sexuality, and the Intersectionality in Public Health." *Culture, Health & Sexuality* 7, no. 6 (Nov.–Dec. 2005): 16–23.

Elford, J., G. Bolding, and L. Sherr. "High-risk Behavior Increases among London Gay Men between 1998 and 2001: What Is the Role of HIV Optimism?" *AIDS* 16 (2002): 1537–44.

Epstein, J. *Altered Conditions: Disease, Medicine and Storytelling.* New York and London: Routledge, 1995.

Epstein, S. "Bodily Differences and Collective Identities: The Politics of Gender and Race in Biomedical Research in the United States." *Body & Society* 10, no. 2–3 (2004): 183–203.

———. *Impure Science: AIDS, Activism, and the Politics of Knowledge.* Berkeley: University of California Press, 1996.

Exner, T. M., S. Hoffman, S. Dworkin, and A. A. Ehrhardt. "Beyond the Male Condom: The Evolution of Gender-Specific HIV Interventions for Women." *Annual Review of Sex Research* 14 (2003): 114–36.

Fassin, D. *When Bodies Remember: Experiences and Politics of AIDS in South Africa.* Berkeley: University of California Press, 2007.

Ferner, R. E. "The Influence of Big Pharma." Editorial in *British Medical Journal* 33 (2006): 857–58.

Flowers, P. "Gay Men and HIV/AIDS Risk Management." *Health* 5, no. 1 (2001): 50–75.

Franklin, S., C. Lury, and J. Stacey. *Global Nature, Global Culture.* London: Sage, 2000.

Fraser, M. "The Ethics of Reality and Virtual Reality: Latour, Facts and Values." *History of the Human Sciences* 19 (2006): 45–72.

———. "Standards, Populations, and Difference." Special issue, *Cultural Critique* (forthcoming).

———. "What Is the Matter of Feminist Criticism." *Economy and Society* 31, no. 4 (2002): 606–25.

Frenkel, L. M., and J. I. Mullins. "Should Patients with Drug-Resistant HIV-1 Continue to Receive Antiretroviral Therapy?" *New England Journal of Medicine* 344, no. 7 (2001): 520–22.

Gates, W. "Bill and Melinda Gates Announce a Commitment to Supporting Microbicide Research." 16th International AIDS Conference, Toronto, Canada, 2006. See http://www.cnn.com/2006/HEALTH/08/16/aids.transmission.cnn/ or http://www.seedmagazine.com/news/2006/08/at_aids_conference_vaccines_ta.php.

Ghosn, J., J. Viard, C. Katlama, M. de Almeida, R. Tubiana, F. Letourneur, L. Aaron, C. M. Giele, R. Maw, C. A. Carne, and B. G. Evans, on behalf of the British Co-operative Clinical Group of the Medical Society for the Study of Venereal Diseases. "Post-exposure Prophylaxis for Non-occupational Exposure to HIV: Current Clinical Practice and Opinions in the UK." *Sexually Transmitted Infections* 78, no. 2 (April 2002): 130–32.

GlaxoSmithKline Web site. http://us.gsk.com/.

Global Microbicide Campaign. *Fact Sheet 4: Gender Equality in AIDS Protection.* 2005.

Gray, R., X. Li, G. Kigozi, D. Serwadda, H. Brahmbhatt, F. Wabwire-Mangen, F. Nalugoda, M. Kiddugavu, N. Sewankambo, and T. Quinn. "Increased Risk of Incident HIV During Pregnancy in Rakai, Uganda: A Prospective Study." *The Lancet* 366, no. 9492 (2005): 1182–88.

Green, R. E., and D. J. Ward. "Let's Call It HIV Infection, Not 'AIDS.'" Poster presented at the 14th International AIDS Conference, AIDS 2002, Barcelona, Spain, 7–12 July 2002.

Grover, J. "OI: Opportunistic Identification, Open Identification, in PWA Portraiture." In *Don't Leave Me This Way: Art in the Age of AIDS*, compiled by Ted Gott. Melbourne: National Gallery of Australia; London and New York: Thames and Hudson, 1994.

Guatelli, J., D. Goff, and N. Van Damme. *Modulation of Viral Assembly and Virion Release by Vpu*. 15th Conference on Retroviruses and Opportunistic Infections, Boston, abstract 104a, 2008.

Halperin, D. *What Do Gay Men Want?: An Essay on Sex, Risk, and Subjectivity*. Ann Arbor: University of Michigan Press, 2007.

Hanson, B. "Bodily Differences and Collective Identities: The Politics of Gender and Race in Biomedical Research in the United States." In *Social Assumptions, Medical Categories*. Greenwich, CT: JAI Press, 1977.

Haraway, D. *Modest_Witness@Second_Millennium: FemaleMan©_MeetsOncoMouse™*. New York and London: Routledge, 1997.

———. *Simians, Cyborgs, and Women: The Reinvention of Nature*. London: Free Association Books, 1991.

———. "Situated Knowledges." In *Feminism and Science*, edited by E. Fox Keller and H. Longino. Oxford: Oxford University Press, 1991.

Haseltine, W. A., and F. Wong-Staal. "The Molecular Biology of the AIDS Virus." *Scientific American* 259, no. 4 (1988): 34–42.

Herzig, R. "On Performance, Productivity, and Vocabularies of Motive in Recent Studies of Science." *Feminist Theory* 5, no. 2 (2004): 127–47.

Hird, M. "Chimerism, Mosaicism and the Cultural Construction of Kinship." *Sexualities* 7, no. 2 (2004): 217–232.

Ho, D. "Time to Hit HIV, Early and Hard." *New England Journal of Medicine* 333, no. 7 (1995): 450–51.

Institute of Science in Society. "Women Confront AIDS in Africa," http://www.i-sis.org.uk/Women_Confront_Aids_in_Africa.php.

Jaffe, H. W., R. O. Valdisseri, and K. M. De Cock. "The Reemerging HIV/AIDS Epidemic in Men Who Have Sex with Men." *Journal of the American Medical Association* 298, no. 20 (2007): 2412–14.

Jintarkanon S., S. Nakapiew, N. Tienudom, P. Suwannawong, and D. Wilson. "Unethical Clinical Trials in Thailand: A Community Response." *The Lancet* 3, no. 65 (7 May 2005): 1617–18.

*Journal of the American Medical Association* 285, no. 1 (3 January 2001): 34.

Kippax, S., and K. Race. "Sustaining Safe Practice: Twenty Years On." *Social Science & Medicine* 57 (2003): 1–12.

Kirby, V. "Human Nature." *Australian Feminist Studies* 14, no. 29 (1999): 19–29.

Lash, S., and C. Lury. *Global Culture Industries: The Mediation of Things*. Cambridge, UK, and Malden, MA: Polity Press, 2007.

Latour, B. "How to Talk About the Body? The Normative Dimension of Science Studies." *Body & Society* 10, no. 2–3 (2004): 205–29.

———. *We Have Never Been Modern*. Trans. C. Porter. Cambridge: Harvard University Press, 1993.

Law, J., and J. Urry. "Enacting the Social." *Economy and Society* 33 (3 August 2004): 390–410.

Lewis, S. UN Special Envoy for HIV/AIDS in Africa, University of Pennsylvania's Summit on Global Issues in Women's Health, Philadelphia, 26 April 2005.

Little, S. J., S. Holte, J. Routy, E. S. Daar, M. Markowitz, A. C. Collier, R. A. Koup, J. W. Mellors, E. Connick, B. Conway, M. Kilby, L. Wang, J. M. Whitcomb, N. S. Hellmann, and D. D. Richman. "Antiretroviral-Drug Resistance among Patients Recently Infected with HIV." *New England Journal of Medicine* 34, no. 6 (8 August 2002): 385–94.

Little, S. "Is Transmitted Drug Resistance in HIV on the Rise?" *British Medical Journal* 322 (2001): 1074–75.

Longino, H. "Subjects, Power, and Knowledge: Description and Prescription in Feminist Philosophies of Science." In *Feminism and Science*, edited by E. Fox Keller and H. Longino. Oxford: Oxford University Press, 1996.

Lury, C. "From Diversity to Heterogeneity: A Feminist Analysis of the Making of Kinds." *Economy and Society* 31, no. 4 (2002): 588–605.

Mackenzie, A. *Transductions: Bodies and Machines at Speed*. London and New York: Continuum, 2002.

McCune, J. M. "The Dynamics of CD4 T-cell Depletion in HIV Disease." *Nature* 410 (2001): 974–79.

McDiarmid, D. "there isn't room for ambiguity." AIDS Action Council of New South Wales, http://www.aidsaction.org.au/content/events/reflections/there_isnt_room_for_ambiguity.php.

Mao, L., J. M. Crawford, H. J. Hospers, G. P. Prestage, A. E. Grulich, J. M. Kaldor, and S. C. Kippax. "'Serosorting' in Casual Anal Sex of HIV-negative Gay Men Is Noteworthy and Is Increasing in Sydney, Australia." *AIDS* 20, no. 8 (12 May 2006): 1204–6.

Merck Web site. http://www.merck.com.

Michael, M. *Technoscience and Everyday Life: The Complex Simplicities of the Mundane*. Berkshire, UK: Open University Press, 2006).

Mitchell, R., and P. Thurtle. *Data Made Flesh*. New York and London: Routledge, 2004.

Mol, A. *The Body Multiple: Ontology in Medical Practice*. Durham, NC: Duke University Press, 2003.

Montaner, S. G., R. Hogg, E. Wood, T. Kerr, M. A. Tyndall, R. Levy, and P. R. Harrigan. "The Case for Expanding Access to Highly Active Antiretroviral Therapy to Curb the Growth of the HIV Epidemic," *The Lancet* 368 (2006): 531–36.

Moynihan, R., I. Heath, and D. Henry. "Selling Sickness: The Pharmaceutical Industry and Disease Mongering." *British Medical Journal* 324 (13 April 2002): 886–91.

Murphy, D. "Risk reduction strategies for anal sex with casual partners." AFAO/NAPWA Education Discussion Paper 2, no. 4, 2000/2001 (2001).

NAM. "Aidsmap: Information on hiv & aids," http://www.aidsmap.com/en/default.asp.

National Health Institutes Web site. http://grants.nih.gov/grants/funding/phs398/instructions2/p2_nih_policy_report_race_ethnicity.htm.

Nguyen, V. "Antiretroviral Globalism, Biopolitics, and Therapeutic Citizenship." In *Global Assemblages: Technology, Politics and Ethics as Anthropological Problems*, edited by Aihwa Ong and Stephen J. Collier. Cambridge, UK, and Malden, MA: Blackwell, 2005.

Novas, C., and N. Rose. "Genetic Risk and the Birth of the Somatic Individual." Special issue, *Economy and Society* 29, no. 4 (2000): 484–513.

Oldani, M. J. "Thick Prescriptions: Toward an Interpretation of Pharmaceutical Sales Practices." *Medical Quarterly Anthropology* 18, no. 3 (September 2004): 325–56.

Palella, F. J., K. M. Dalaney, A. C. Moorman, et al. "Declining Morbidity and Mortality among Patients with Advanced Human Immunodeficiency Virus Infection." *New England Journal of Medicine* 338 (1998): 853–60.

Patton, C. *Globalizing AIDS*. Minneapolis: University of Minnesota Press, 2002.

———. *Inventing AIDS*. New York and London: Routledge, 1990.

Persson, A., E. Wakeford, and K. Race. "HIV Health in Context: Negotiating Medical Technology and Lived Experience." *Health: An Interdisciplinary Journal for the Social Study of Health, Illness and Medicine* 7 (2003): 397–415.

Persson, A. "Incorporating Pharmakon: HIV, Medicine, and Body Shape Change." *Body & Society* 10, no. 4 (2004): 45–67.

Picker, L. J., and D. I. Watkins. "HIV Pathogenesis: The First Cut Is the Deepest." *Nature Immunology* 6, no. 5 (2005): 430–32.

*Positive Nation* 64 (2001): 35.

*Positive Nation Treatment News* 14 (March 2001): 35.

Quinn, T. C., M. J. Wawer, N. Sewankambo, D. Serwadda, Li Chuanjun, F. Wabwire-Mangen, M. O. Meehan, T. Lutalo, and R. H. Gray. "Viral Load and Heterosexual Transmission of Human Immunodeficiency Virus Type I." *New England Journal of Medicine* 342 (2000): 921–29.

Rabinow, P. "Artificiality and Enlightenment: From Sociobiology to Biosociality." In *Essays on the Anthropology of Reason*. Princeton, NJ: Princeton University Press, 1996.

Race, K. "Revaluation of Risk among Gay Men." *AIDS Education and Prevention* 4 (2003): 369–81.

Race, K. "The Undetectable Crisis: Changing Technologies of Risk." *Sexualities* 4, no. 2 (2001): 167–89.

Race, K., and Wakeford, E. "Dosing on Time: Developing Adherent Practice with Highly Active Anti-retroviral Therapy." *Culture, Health & Sexuality* 2, no. 2 (2000): 213–228.

Reardon, J. "Decoding Race and Human Difference in a Genomic Age." *differences: A Journal of Feminist Cultural Studies* 15, no. 3 (2004): 38–65.

Reardon, J., B. Dunklee, and K. Wentworth. "Race and Crisis." *Social Science Research Forum,* 1 June 2005, htttp://raceandgenomics.ssrc.org/Reardon/pf.

Reuters NewMedia, "Glaxo AIDS Drug Less Effective Than Others: Trial." 12 March 2003, http://ww2.aegis.org/news/re/2003/RE030309.html.

Richens, J., S. G. Edwards, and S. T. Sadiq. "Can the Promotion of Post-exposure Prophylaxis Following Sexual Exposure to HIV (PEPSE) Cause Harm?" *Sexually Transmitted Infections* 81 (2005): 190–91.

Ridge, D. T. "'It Was an Incredible Thrill': The Social Meanings and Dynamics of Younger Gay Men's Experiences of Barebacking in Melbourne." *Sexualities* 7, no. 3 (2004): 259–79.

Risch, N., E. Burchard, E. Ziv, and H. Tang. "Categorization of Humans in Biomedical Research: Genes, Race and Disease." *Genome Biology* 3, no. 7 (2002): comment 2007.1–2007.12.

Rose, N., and C. Novas. "Biological Citizenship." In *Global Assemblages: Technology, Politics and Ethics as Anthropological Problems,* edited by Aihwa Ong and Stephen Collier, 439–63. Oxford: Blackwell, 2005.

Rosengarten, M., K. Race, and S. Kippax. "'Touch Wood, Everything Will Be OK': Gay Men's Understandings of Clinical Markers in Sexual Practise." *Monograph 7/2000* Sydney: National Centre in HIV Social Research, 2000.

Rosengarten, M., J. Imrie, P. Flowers, M. D. Davis, and G. J. Hart. "After the Euphoria: HIV Medical Technologies from the Perspective of Clinicians." *Sociology of Health and Illness* 26, no. 5 (2004): 575–96.

Schapiro, J. "Understanding Protease Inhibitor Potency: The Intersection of Exposure, Efficacy, and Resistance." *The AIDS Reader* 1, no. 6 (2001): 311–15.

Sheon, N., and M. G. Crosby. "Ambivalent Tales of HIV Disclosure in San Francisco." *Social Science & Medicine* 58 (2004): 2105–18.

Smith, R. "Medical Journals and Pharmaceutical Companies: Uneasy Bedfellows." *British Medical Journal* 326 (2003): 1202–5.

Spurgeon, D. "Companies May Face Tighter Regulation over Promoting Drugs." *British Medical Journal* 329 (2004): 998.

Stephenson, J. M., J. Imrie, M. M. D. Davis, C. Mercer, S. Black, A. J. Copas, G. J. Hart, O. R. Davidson and I. G. Williams. "Is Use of Antiretroviral Therapy among Homosexual Men Associated with Increased Risk of Transmission of

HIV Infection?" *Sexually Transmitted Infections* 79 (2003): 7–10.

Sterling, T. R., D. Vlahov, J. Astemborski, D. R. Hoover, J. B. Margolick, and T. C. Quinn. "Initial Plasma HIV-1 RNA Levels and Progression to AIDS in Women and Men." *New England Journal of Medicine* 344, no. 10 (2001): 720–25.

Treichler, P. A. "AIDS, Homophobia and Biomedical Discourse: An Epidemic of Signification." *October* 43 (1987): 31–70.

———. *How to Have Theory in an Epidemic: Cultural Chronicles of AIDS.* Durham, NC: Duke University Press, 1999.

True Vision. "Dying for Drugs," directed by Brian Edwards, aired on UK Channel 4 television, April 2003.

UK Collaborative Group on Monitoring the Transmission of HIV Drug Resistance. "Analysis of Prevalence of HIV-1 Drug Resistance in Primary Infections in the United Kingdom." *British Medical Journal* 322 (2007): 1087–88.

Valdiserri, R. O. "Mapping the Roots of HIV/AIDS Complacency: Implications for Program and Policy Development." *AIDS Education and Prevention* 16, no. 5 (2004): 426–39.

Van de Ven, P., G. Prestage, J. Crawford, A. Grulich, and S. Kippax. "Sexual Risk Behaviour Increases and Is Associated with HIV Treatment Optimism among HIV-negative and HIV-positive Gay Men in Sydney over the Four-year Period to February 2000." *AIDS* 14 (2000): 2952–53.

Van de Ven, P., J. Crawford, S. Kippax, S. Knox, G. Prestage. "A Scale of Optimism-Scepticism in the Context of HIV Treatments." *AIDS Care* 12 (2000): 171–76.

Van de Ven, P., S. Kippax, J. Crawford, P. Rawstorne, G. Prestage, A. Grulich, and D. Murphy. "In a Minority of Gay Men, Sexual Risk Practice Indicates Strategic Positioning for Perceived Risk Reduction Rather than Unbridled Sex." *AIDS Care* 14 (2002): 471–80.

Vernazza, P., B. Hirschel, E. Bernasconi, and M. Flepp. "Les personnes sèropositives ne souffrant d'aucune autre MST et suivant un traitement antirètroviral efficace ne transmettent pas le VIH par voie sexuelle." *Bulletin des mèdecins suisses* 89, no. 5 (2008).

Wagner, G. "Does Discontinuing the Use of Pill Boxes to Facilitate Electronic Monitoring Impede Adherence?" *International Journal of STD and AIDS* 14, no. 1 (2003): 64–65.

Wainberg, M. A., and G. Friedland. "Public Health Implications of Antiretroviral Therapy and HIV Drug Resistance." *Journal of the American Medical Association* 279, no. 24 (1998): 1977–83.

Waldby, C. *Visible Human Project: Informatic Bodies and Posthuman Medicine.* New York and London: Routledge, 2000.

Waldo, C. R., R. D. Stall, and T. J. Coates. "Is Offering Post-exposure Prevention for Sexual Exposures to HIV Related to Sexual Risk Behavior in Gay Men?" *AIDS* 14, no. 8 (2000): 1035–39.

Watney, S. "The Spectacle of AIDS." In *The Lesbian and Gay Studies Reader,* edited by Henry Abelove, Michële Aina Barale, and David M. Halperin. New York and London: Routledge, 1993.

Weiss, R. "Gulliver's Travels in HIVland." *Nature* 410 (2001): 963–67.

Whitehead, A. N. *Process and Reality.* Edited by David Ray Griffin and Donald W. Sherburne. New York and London: Free Press, 1978.

Whitehead, A. N. *Science and the Modern World.* London: Free Association Books, 1985.

Willems, D. "Inhaling Drugs and Making Worlds: The Proliferation of Lungs and Asthmas." In *Differences in Medicine,* edited by Marc Berg and Annemarie Mol. Durham, NC: Duke University Press, 1998.

Winkler, C., Ping An, and S. J. O'Brien. "Patterns of Ethnic Diversity among the Genes that Influence AIDS." *Human Molecular Genetics* 13, Review Issue 1 (2004): R9–R19.

# Index

99; processual ontology of race in, 88–93, 126n17; the "prototypical human individual," 100; relational conceptions of gender in, 95–98; social-political constructs of, 83–85, 88–96, 125n3; studies of genetic variability in, 85–86; in variations in viral load measures, 90–91, 94–95; in women's vulnerability to HIV, 82, 87–88, 95, 126n11

hybrid forum, 12–13, 50–53; conflicts of interest in, 50–51; of marketing, 37–39, 44; of media coverage, 44–45; pharmaceutical company's orchestration of, 54–57, 119nn25–27; of prevention messages, 14; traffic in, 55–57

iatrogenic disease. *See* side effects of ARVs

imagination, 12, 27; contribution to knowledge by, 20–21; in HIV intervention, 24–25, 34; pre-existent presence of, 33–35

individual genetic essence, 99

"Influence of CCR5 Promoter Haplotypes on AIDS Progression in African-Americans" (An et al.), 88–90

information, 4–6, 16–17, 110–11nn9–10; informed matter of the molecule, 14, 62–63, 73, 80–81; mediation of the biological with, 13–14, 74–76, 81, 101–8, 124nn40–41. *See also* risk calculations; science

"Initial Plasma HIV-1 RNA Levels and Progression to AIDS in Women and Men" (Sterling et al.), 94

intersexuality, 97–98, 129n39

intervention, 6–17; activism for improvements in, 36–39, 57–58, 108; "better biology" in, 108; CD4 T-cell counts in, 43, 118n13, 127n31;

128n1; economics of, 3–4, 16, 57–58, 109n4, 113n40, 120n41; full-treatment access in, 109n4; imagination in, 24–25, 34; implications for prevention of, 59–60; male-centered approach of, 87; as performative process, 9–11, 21–25, 33, 34, 102, 106; pre-ARV cultural interventions, 15–16; separation of "human-ness" from, 53, 104–5. *See also* antiretroviral drugs (ARVs); human host factors

*Inventing AIDS* (Patton), 115n33

Johnson, Margaret, 49–50, 119n25

*Journal of the American Medical Association (JAMA)*, 47–48

Kaposi's sarcoma, 66–68

Keogh, Peter, 124n45

Kippax, Susan, 72; on mismatches, 78; on prevention strategies, 122n30; on treatment optimism and risk, 60, 73, 121n8

Kirby, Vicki, 23–24, 115n27

Lamivudine (3TC), 40, 51, 56

language. *See* textual expression

Lash, Scott, 106–7

Latour, Bruno, 10–11, 22, 98–99, 104–5

Law, John, 22, 77, 79, 105–6

lifestyle impact of ARVs, 16–17, 55, 57, 103, 120n40. *See also* side effects of ARVs

lipodistrophy/lipoatrophy, 18

Lury, Celia, 105–7, 129n9

marketing of pharmaceuticals: company orchestration of, 54–56, 119nn25–27; consumer self-identification in, 43; creation of HIV-positive consumers, 53; restrictions on, 40, 118n11, 119n28; through media coverage,

RA
643
.8
.R67
2009